Heart Beats

Heart Beats

REAL PATIENTS REAL STORIES

• • •

Evelyn Lawson-Jonsson RN BSN

Copyright © 2012 Evelyn Lawson-Jonsson RN BSN

ISBN-13: 9781530470525
ISBN-10: 1530470528

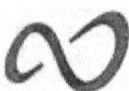

First published by
INFINITY PUBLISHING
1094 New DeHaven Street, Suite 100
West Conshohocken, PA 19428-2713

Dedication

*In loving memory
To my courageous mother, Eugenia Scott, a teacher par excelence*

● ● ●

Preface

● ● ●

The Florence Nightingale Pledge's final lines are:
"...With loyalty will I endeavor to aid the physician in his work and
to devote myself to the welfare of those committed to my care."
Our nursing class solemnly repeated these words at the
beginning of our graduation ceremony.

The guest speaker said the world awaited us,
a heady and scary thought.
One I don't think any of us felt quite ready for.
Much has changed since graduation,
but not the commitment we nurses have to our patients.

Married and (slightly) pregnant at graduation,
I went to work on the pediatric unit
at our University Hospital.
A couple of months later, after passing
State boards, I was hired
at the small community hospital
where this book begins...

...*Most patients* we encounter become the white noise in which we practice our profession. Some patients stand in sharp relief, forming memories we carry throughout our lives. *These are their stories...*

Table of Contents

Tammy

• • •

Tammy

● ● ●

7:30 P.M. MOANS AND SHARP sighs told me my patient was arriving by gurney from the Emergency Room (ER), a 16-year-old girl, Tammy, with acute abdominal pain of unknown origin. I went to help the orderly and nurses' aide transfer her to the bed. Her parents had trailed behind, worried into silence. Even though we were moving her as carefully as possible, she still let out a yelp of pain. After getting her settled, the aide stayed to do the admitting vital signs, her parents hovering near her bedside. Checking the ER record, I noted that she had been given a pain shot just prior to her transfer to our floor. Assuring her that she would feel much better after the medication took effect, I left, promising to check back with her in a few minutes to make sure it had eased her pain.

Out of nursing school for just a couple of months, I had gone to work in our small community hospital. Having oriented to several units, I had not yet been assigned a permanent position. This left me feeling part of nothing and longing for my nursing school days. On this day--just my third day on this surgical unit--the head nurse, Judy, assigned me to be a team leader for half the patients! The first two days I had followed her around as she oriented me. I was excited and scared at the same time, hoping my nursing skill would meet the challenge.

When I graduated all nurses wore white from top to bottom, and the dress code included a nurse's cap. At this particular hospital, that obviously hadn't heard of "women's lib," I learned that nurses stood to give their chair to the doctors, pulled the charts for the doctors, got them coffee. "Doctor will see you now" seemed like announcing an audience with the pope or giving the patient the opportunity to be seen by some kind of deity. Nurses did not question doctors. Doctors questioned nurses, and especially those at the bottom of the hierarchy, where I stood.

At the nurse's station Tammy's surgeon, Dr. Risner, sat finishing his admitting orders. With a quick turn on his heels he headed off down the hall at a fast clip, saying over his shoulder that he would see Tammy in the morning to reevaluate her situation before his surgeries.

The paging system interrupted the flow of the unit by announcing, in a moderately irritating, mechanical sounding voice, at a volume too loud to ignore, that visiting hours were over. In those days it wasn't a suggestion; it was a command. I felt sure Tammy's parents would be obeying reluctantly.

On my patient rounds, I went to see Tammy first. Her face was twisted with pain. She had not responded well to that first pain shot given to her in the ER. I assured her the doctor would be called right away. Hurrying back to the nurse's station, I felt thankful to see Judy charting. Sitting down beside her, I shared my concerns about Tammy. She just raised her eyebrows and said in an authoritative voice, "I have worked with Dr. Risner for many years now, and he really doesn't appreciate unwarranted phone calls. Why don't you give Tammy more time to settle down, recheck her in a half-hour, before you even *think* about calling the doctor?" Certainly not the response I expected. I thought she'd at least come with me to check Tammy.

Maybe I was just too new to know better, or too young to listen, but when Judy headed down the hall, I picked up the telephone and called the doctor anyway. Just like she said, Dr. Risner was unimpressed with my unsolicited update, and let me know in CAPITAL letters--reminding me that Tammy *had* been admitted for *abdominal pain*. He did, however, increase Tammy's Demerol order to 75-100 mg every 3-4 hours, with a STAT dose of an additional 50 mg. Before hanging up, Dr. Risner emphasized that he would see her *in the morning*!

Even with the additional injection, an hour later Tammy was in a fetal position, facing the window. When I asked about her pain, in a quiet voice she said it hurt a little less if she stayed on her side and didn't move. Two shots for pain in two hours, and she felt only *marginally* better? Yet, this time, when I shared my continuing concern with Judy, she shrugged it off saying, "This is probably just a hysterical teenage girl's response to a little pain."

What a dilemma! It seemed to me that Tammy really *had* acute abdominal pain, unrelieved by the pain medications she had already been given--but maybe I was wrong. What if I wasn't? I started to dial her doctor's number but clicked the receiver down before it rang. By then it was almost 10 p.m. and the next shift would be there within the hour. It was tempting to leave her unresolved pain issue for them to deal with. That didn't seem right either. I felt compelled to call her doctor again, knowing Dr. Risner would certainly question my sanity and inexperience and do it all again in capital letters--with a few explicatives thrown in for good measure. During my years doing clinical rotations in nursing school, I had never heard a doctor yell. I certainly wasn't looking forward to hearing this doctor yell at me again!

My heart raced as I dialed his number a second time. Should I have listened to Judy? This time I will probably be waking him up for sure, yet I just couldn't put the receiver down. When he came on the line, I got what I expected: disbelief that he was being bothered again and another tirade of angry words. After Dr. Risner calmed down a little, he finally consented to come in. I felt rung-out, exhausted. Now I sat waiting to hear his dreaded footsteps coming down the darkened hallway. What if I had called him for nothing? Could this be my last day here? Could I be fired for this? What a dreadful thought!

Unfortunately when Dr. Risner arrived, his mood had not improved. Clipped questions and orders confirmed his continued anger at being called out so late. However, after examining Tammy, he did order STAT lab work. When the results came back, he had us prepare Tammy for an immediate exploratory operation. Next, he sat down to call her parents with his findings. By the time Tammy was wheeled off to surgery, the p.m. shift had bled over onto the night shift and I was still there catching up on charting for my other patients.

When I finally walked out the door, I was dazed from the confrontations and still concerned about Tammy. What will they find in surgery? Nothing? Or maybe something really bad? How awkward will it be to see Dr. Risner again? What will tomorrow bring? Will I still be working with Judy? Would they transfer me to another unit, or even fire me? After all, I hadn't followed my head nurse's directions. Ugh!

The next day I found out Tammy's abdominal pain had been caused by an undiagnosed ectopic pregnancy, a life-threatening condition that only the surgery could have remedied. At that moment, I knew that the most important responsibility I would ever have as a nurse would be as an advocate for my patient, *regardless* of the consequences. And, Dr. Risner? He came by while I was charting later that afternoon. I looked up, waiting for him to speak. Was he still mad? When he said, "Good call," I let out the breath I did not know I was holding and watched dumbfounded as he headed down the hall.

Observing in the ER

• • •

Observing in the ER

● ● ●

MY EXCITEMENT TO START A week of observation in the ER was quickly drained away when I met the head nurse in charge. She stood tall, straight, and stiffly starched. Her demeanor reeked of the military and I felt intimidated. This week of observation was not going to be a cozy little chat with her sharing information about *her* Emergency Room. She would dictate; I would listen.

Efficiently and methodically, "Miss Fastidious" ran the department like a ship: "a place for everything and everything in its place" at all times. Stainless steel surfaces gleamed. When there were no patients to care for, she checked and rechecked her supplies. It seemed a little obsessive to me.

On my last day of observation, ambulances brought in three seriously injured family members who had been involved in a single car accident. From the police and ambulance driver we learned that the father had somehow lost control and the car glanced off a telephone pole before rolling down a steep embankment.

The father was barely conscious and bleeding profusely from his multiple head injuries, complicated by crushing injuries to his chest from being pinned by the steering wheel. His wife, wearing no seat belt, had been thrown from the car, probably saving her life as the passenger side of the car had been completely crushed. On arrival her vital signs were unstable and she was unresponsive, even to painful stimuli. The multiple layers of gaze bandages applied to her head and neck at the scene were soaked with bright red blood. Her left leg had been splinted.

Their fourteen-year-old daughter was alert and insistently asking about her parents. She was given sketchy information, but it was enough to satisfy her panicky concerns. She had sustained a compound fracture (bones coming through the skin) of her left forearm and suffered multiple lacerations and contusions.

I heard the overhead speakers urgently summoning medical and nursing staff to the ER. Soon doctors and nurses came rushing to assist these critically injured patients. The department vibrated with intense activity. "Miss Fastidious" knew exactly where to find the supplies needed to treat each patient.

The mother was stabilized and immediately transferred per ambulance to a larger hospital that provided neurological care. The father's chest wound required the placement of a chest tube to improve his respiratory status by allowing his collapsed lung to re-inflate. Two units of O-Negative blood were pumped through the IV to compensate for the copious amounts of blood he had lost. Lacerations were quickly sutured so he could be transferred to ICU for further observation and care. The daughter's lacerations were sutured and she was sent to surgery for an emergency "open reduction" of her fractured right arm.

It was amazing to see that instead of chaos, total efficiency reigned. The policies and procedures of "Miss Fastidious" proved invaluable.

The Gun Shot Patient

• • •

The Gun Shot Patient

• • •

LATER THAT MONTH, THE SUPERVISOR sent me to help with a full Emergency Room. Stepping off the elevator, I could see through the partially open staff door the team frantically working over a patient with his boots still on. Not a good sign. An anxious, middle-aged couple paced in the area just outside the door. Slipping by them, I entered the drama, drawn like a moth to the light.

The outcome for the patient: uncertain. The victim: a fifteen-year-old boy. He had been accidentally shot in the head while loading a gun with his friend. The details didn't matter. All that mattered was that this teenager receive the best care available, and as quickly as possible. A palpable intensity pervaded the air as the ER team fought for a life too young to perish. For over an hour the team endeavored to save him, but in the end all their efforts couldn't reverse the damage done by one senseless mistake.

Later, I heard the wails of the parents, different from any sound I had ever heard, after they had been informed of their son's tragic outcome. Even after the Chaplain eased them into the elevator, to take them up to the chapel, the sounds of their cries muffled by closed doors and the upward assent of the elevator were painful to hear and impossible not to feel. The loss, so large and irrevocable, hung in the air. The vacuum left from the energy expended fighting for this young man's life sucked at the bone marrow of those of us left to clean up the vainly used supplies and prepare for the next opportunity to cheat death.

Ruben

· · ·

Ruben

● ● ●

THEY MUST HAVE BEEN DESPERATE for someone to cover ER. Why else would the Supervisor ask me to fill in for a sick nurse? My qualifications were really slim. Having recently graduated from a nursing school that didn't even have an ER rotation, and having spent only one week of *observation* in the hospital's ER, this request took me totally off guard.

Added to my lack of experience was the fact that I was six months pregnant, stood five feet two inches tall and weighed one hundred ten pounds. It seemed obvious; she had no better choice. Being new I felt obligated to help. When I told her I certainly didn't relish the idea of working alone, the Supervisor assured me she would come help me immediately, if needed. With that assurance, I reluctantly consented.

A few easily handled cases came in: a simple closed arm fracture needing casting, sutures for a laceration from a bicycle rollover, a child with a high fever. Then the department sat totally empty. To pass the time, I cleaned and restocked the suites as part of my responsibilities and spot mopped the floor.

The Supervisor relieved me for supper between seven and seven-thirty. When I got back, a patient being admitted for chest pain, lay on a gurney ready to be transferred to ICU. An orderly stood by as the Supervisor quickly finished charting. Soon they left together, leaving me alone in the department. With nothing else to do I picked up one of those "special" policy and procedure manuals to read and soon became bored. "These books would make excellent sleep aides," I thought irreverently.

About that time a sleazily dressed, unruly young man came stumbling through the doors supported by two equally skuzzy looking friends. Bleeding heavily from a gash on his head, he and his friends reeked of booze. My patient, apparently more inebriated than his friends, needed their assistance to even get up onto the gurney. He sat on the edge looking down, muttering a multitude of swear words, and dripping blood on his filthy shoes *and* the floor I had just finished mopping. After a lot of coaching, he finally lay back and I grabbed some 4x4's and applied pressure to stop the bleeding, the discomfort making him squirm.

Why I thought this case could be handled by one person, let alone me, only testifies to my naïveté about how fast a situation can go from seemingly manageable to totally out of control. I would soon learn. His friends supplied his name, Ruben, and age, nineteen, for the admitting form but no address, last name or phone number. The information his friends gave about his injury and how it occurred was vague, and reluctantly supplied. When the on-call doctor arrived, he would probably succeed in getting answers to these questions as he took the History and Physical. Now all I needed was Ruben's signature on the admission form.

Angry and agitated, he began to thrash around. Thankfully I had put both side rails up, but as Ruben continued thrashing, I rapidly became concerned that he might just come over the top. Having never dealt with an inebriated patient and unaware of the strength a person could muster in this condition, I stepped up on the little metal stool to get his signature. At this point he started yelling in a slurred voice, "Not signin' nothin'" over and over again, the volume getting louder each time he repeated it. In retrospect, that moment would have been a perfect time for me to get out of Ruben's range and call for help. The rules were clear. I needed to get the patient's signature on the admitting form *before* calling the doctor. Being new, I was determined to do it right. However, that rule probably didn't mean at the risk of life and limb.

Next, Ruben did try to climb over the rails. Soon I found myself stretched out across him trying to reach a needed hand restraint on the opposite rail, but then my feet slipped off the stool leaving me teetering on my baby-filled tummy across Ruben's abdomen. Sometimes in adrenaline-charged moments like this, everything seems to slow down. Little things are noticed: the blood splatters congealing on the beige-spotted linoleum squares on the opposite side of the gurney or the ubiquitous hospital-green walls that blurred as they tilted by in my peripheral vision. In the midst of this drama I made a mental note to be sure to mop up that blood. No doubt "Miss Fastidious" would notice my lapse. As waves of nausea rolled over me, the thought occurred to me to suggest they paint those sickening green walls a different color. Maybe a light cream?

Fortunately, Ruben's friends came to my rescue. Maybe the cute little white uniform dresses that I usually wore weren't appropriate for the ER; especially since mine had now worked its way up farther than I care to say. Anyway, Ruben's friends held onto him and somehow helped me slip back down onto the stool. As they struggled with Ruben, I ran to the emergency bell to summon help.

True to her word, the Supervisor, along with two orderlies, arrived in rapid succession and properly restrained Ruben. The on-call doctor followed on their heels and after hearing the story, decided to check me out first to make sure being roughed-up had only hurt my dignity and not my baby. Then the Supervisor insisted on calling my husband to come pick me up. I felt totally exhausted after the adrenaline rush and readily agreed. Ruben's friends made a quick exit just prior to the arrival of two police officers that stood by as the doctor finished suturing his gash. Then they escorted Ruben off to jail. My husband arrived to take me home. I felt shaken but wiser, and not at all bad about managing to get out of mopping that floor once more.

Orienting to the Newborn Nursery

• • •

Orienting to the Newborn Nursery

● ● ●

THE OB DEPARTMENT, OFTEN CALLED the "Happy Unit," is a world unto itself, consisting of Labor and Delivery, Postpartum, and the Nursery. Nurses seemed to either love the department or hate it, with not much room in between. I loved it, having worked part-time in the Nursery during my senior year in nursing school.

The first thing we were required to do, before entering the Nursery was to scrub our hands and arms up to the elbows, turning them red with irritation. Rough sterile towels were provided for drying. If we left the Nursery, we had to repeat the above process before re-entering this "sacred" space. After several trips out it seemed that there couldn't be any skin left to be scrubbed off. Because of this, trips outside the Nursery were carefully planned and kept to a minimum.

Basically, we cared for healthy newborns and a few stable, premature infants, who stayed with us while they gained enough weight to go home. As a small community hospital, mothers with high-risk pregnancies or infants born needing Neonatal Intensive Care were sent on to larger hospitals with specialty units to handle such complications.

The Labor and Delivery Room nurses brought newborns to us, swaddled in receiving blankets. After being weighed and measured, they were given their first baths. Most of the babies were quite vocal about not wanting to be disturbed by our routines. Others just gazed at us or looked around the room, seemingly content with whatever needed to be done.

As soon as possible newborns were taken to their mother's room for bonding time. What a privilege for us to be part of the team welcoming these precious babies into the world. I could envision myself applying for an opening in the Nursery, even knowing that openings were few and far between.

Katie

• • •

Katie

● ● ●

A BABY GIRL WAS BORN too soon, weighing only a few ounces over three pounds. Breathing well on her own meant she would be kept in our Nursery until she gained enough weight to be discharged. The birth mother had chosen to adopt her to a two-parent home. Though I had never met her, my heart went out to her. Now, seven months pregnant, I wondered how she made such a courageous decision.

Social Services contacted the adoptive family soon after the baby girl arrived. The Berkleys were surprised to get this call two months earlier than expected--excited but concerned about her condition. They were reassured to hear that even though she was tiny, she was breathing on her own and the pediatrician had carefully examined her and reported that she was doing well, so far. The "primi" (born prematurely) would be kept in an isolette to keep her from expending energy generating warmth that she needed to use to gain weight.

The adoptive couple excitedly said they would be on the road within just a few minutes. The drive took over an hour at best on a good day through Southern California traffic. As soon as they arrived and looked at the skinny little bit of life that would be theirs, tears trickled down their faces. "She is so beautiful." "Look at her tiny fingers." On and on and on... the words, a part of the welcoming process, brought us into their joy as well. Soon they were talking about names, finally announcing she would be called Katie Anne. Katie, for her paternal grandmother, and Anne, her adoptive mother's first name.

During the six weeks in which Katie "boarded" in our nursery, her parents drove down each evening just to look through the window at their baby. Parents were not allowed in nurseries in those days. If bonding with a newborn could happen through a thick glass window, it surely did for this precious baby and her adoptive family. Sometimes Katie slept through their entire visit, and the Berkleys seemed just as pleased as when she yawned, stretched, opened her eyes, and kicked her legs as she reached for the sky. She gained weight steadily, first from feedings through an n/g tube into her tiny tummy. After about a month, she began sucking on the tube, an indication that she had developed a sucking reflex. Soon after that the pediatrician started her on formula using a "primi" nipple. With the bottle feedings, Katie continuing to gain weight until she finally tipped the scale at five pounds and was ready for discharge.

This extended time allowed us to bond with Katie, and with her adoptive parents as well. Understandably, it was a bittersweet day when we said farewell, bundling her off with her new family. What a lucky little girl. What lucky parents. A new little family formed. And lucky us, who got to watch it all come together, through the window glass of our Nursery.

Orienting to Labor and Delivery

• • •

Orienting to Labor and Delivery

• • •

IN NURSING SCHOOL MY OB rotation amounted to a few weeks observing and caring for several patients in labor. Our clinical hours were from eight in the morning until noon. Each day of clinical I hoped I could be present for one of the births. But, none of the babies cooperated during my rotation. I felt I had missed the crowning event (pun intended).

That little experience from nursing school left me wanting more, and now my opportunity had arrived. I patiently waded though my orientation to the Postpartum Unit. It was okay taking care of post partum mothers, but I wanted to be downstairs in Labor and Delivery, where the "action" happened.

Our small hospital had only two delivery rooms and three labor rooms. Fathers were allowed in the labor rooms, but our hospital, like many of the hospitals at that time, had not started letting them in the delivery rooms. Most of the patient's labor experiences fell within a normal range. However some were very short, the patient delivering within an hour or so of admission. Occasionally, if a labor became unusually long and/ or particularly difficult, the patient went upstairs for X-rays. (Sonogram technology had not reached our small x-ray department). A fetal monitor, which could be attached to the baby's head during labor, had just been purchased, but used only if there were signs of fetal distress.

Checking cervical dilation and palpating the swollen abdomen determined the progress of labor and the fetal presentation. The mother's abdomen remained a mystery to me. I hadn't yet learned to tell whether the head was up or down. With small hands and short fingers, it was difficult for me to determine the centimeters the cervix had dilated until late in the labor, when the baby's head, most often the presenting part, was within my reach. It was disappointing to realize that Labor and Delivery would probably not be a suitable career path for me.

The baby's status was monitored by frequent checks of the heart rate with a stethoscope. Learning to locate and count the baby's very fast and faint pulse, while ignoring the mother's dominant heart sounds, challenged me. Thankfully, I eventually learned to do that competently.

The doctors checked on their patients soon after admission, and then monitored the patient's progress several times during labor. Learning when to call the doctors for a delivery (definitely an art, not a science) takes a lot of experience to master. Even when mastered, babies can be quite cunning, choosing to make sudden, unanticipated arrival. The staff is left floundering: trying to get the doctor, moving the mother to the delivery room, and making sure the supplies were available and out, all at the same time. Some babies skipped all these delivery room activities and made unplanned arrivals in the labor room.

Because I was still orienting, an experienced nurse would verify for me when to call the doctor for my patient. There were three doctors who did most of the deliveries, and none of them wanted to arrive in the department and be kept waiting because an inexperienced nurse made the decision to call too soon.

One evening on my shift, we had two patients in labor while both of the delivery rooms were in use, a very active time for our small unit with limited staffing. Corrina was in a well-established labor with her third baby. With two boys at home she definitely planned to have a girl this time. I had spent several hours of nervous hovering and monitoring, while Corrina described her baby girl's nursery in detail. Finally, it seemed to me that her doctor should be called. I went looking for an available nurse for a second opinion. No one had time to check my patient's progress so the charge nurse authorized me to go ahead and call her doctor myself. This was scary for me, but since there wasn't another option, I paged his number.

He must have been in the doctor's lounge because he walked through the swinging doors in less than five minutes. My heart thumped in my chest as he impatiently stood over me as I struggled to get Corrina on the gurney, not even offering to help. When we arrived in the delivery room, the nurses had just finished cleaning up from the last delivery and were, thankfully, scurrying around preparing the suite for my patient. As we were getting her draped and making her as comfortable as possible with her feet in the stirrups, the doctor started yelling, "Why didn't you call me when you were actually ready? You have wasted ten minutes of my time!" I felt sorry for my patient; after all, she had been the one laboring for several hours. Fortunately, her delivery was quick and routine. Unfortunately the baby she delivered turned out to be a third boy. The mother, who had told us all along she wanted a girl, started swearing! Now we had an upset doctor and a disappointed mother! What happened to "The Happy Unit" I had been told about?

Teresa

• • •

Teresa

• • •

Teresa arrived by wheelchair in our Labor and Delivery Department, in the second stage of labor with regular contractions and an anxious, solicitous husband. They came with a Lamaze Childbirth Manual, extra pillows, other recommended items, and the wide-eyed look of first-time parents.

She was petite except for an expanded midsection. Her husband, Mark, tall and gangly, stood anxious by her bed, ready to help in any way possible. Teresa's vital signs were normal and the baby's heart rate in the expected range. Within the hour all that would change.

The situation soon shifted from an expected routine delivery to an emergency C-Section, the baby's heart rate dropping precipitously with each contraction. We quickly transferred Teresa to a gurney, rushed her to the elevator and up to OR. She signed the surgical consent form with one hand, holding tightly to Mark's hand with the other. He tried to reassure her as fear and anxiety raced across his face. At the door he squeezed her hand, gave her a kiss, and promised to say a prayer for her and their baby.

We entered the OR suite where preparations were in high gear, instruments jangling as they were tossed on the sterile draped trays. The anesthesiologist sat adjusting his equipment, as the obstetrician pushed his arms through the sleeves of the waiting gown and into sterile gloves which the nurse held for him. I was to take the baby from the doctor's hands, place it in the warm bassinet, and provide the initial care for the baby. I was excited!

Teresa was pulled onto the table using the sheets underneath her. The scrub nurses immediately began preparing her lower abdomen for a "bikini line" incision as the anesthesiologist started the IV and began preparing sedation medications for her. Teresa was quickly turned on her side for a spinal anesthetic so she could be awake for the birth of her baby.

This was my first time observing a C-Section. My eyes were riveted to the surgical site, amazed to see how quickly and efficiently the obstetrician worked, knowing the baby's life depended on it. Within just two or three minutes, he reached in and lifted out a glistening, blue-tinged baby, the umbilical cord wrapped twice around its neck! Immediately he removed the cord from the baby's neck, suctioned its mouth, and rubbed its tiny body with his hands. A hush of anticipation, tinged with fragments of fear, accompanies any delivery until the baby's first cry is heard. He continued rubbing the baby's back until it finally let out cry. A collective sigh of relief swept silently through the room. Next, the doctor clamped and cut the cord and announced that the baby was a girl.

I now felt frightened as I stood holding a receiving blanket, hoping the slippery baby wouldn't land on the floor when the doctor handed the baby to me. I will never forget the awe of that moment when the weight of her tiny body transferred from the doctor's hands into mine. I quickly put her in our bassinet, used the bulb syringe to clear her airway, and gently wiped the bloody mucus from her face. Then I put silver nitrate drops in her eyes to prevent infection. After putting an identification bracelet on her tiny arm, the scrub nurse took the mother's bracelet and placed it on Teresa's wrist. The baby, now wrapped in a fresh pink (naturally) receiving blanket, was ready to be shown to her anxiously awaiting mother. With Teresa's arms secured by the anesthesiologist for her IV's, I held her baby close to her face. She smiled and gave her a first kiss, whispering, "Hello, my precious Hope." A smile of sweet satisfaction swept across her face. Then anesthetic medications were added to her IV solution and she drifted off to sleep, oblivious to the rest of the procedure.

Placing Hope back in the heated bassinet, I tucked an extra blanket around her, turned my back to open the swinging doors, and pushed her out to the area where Hope's father waited anxiously. The new father's eyes asked how Teresa was doing, and I assured him that everything had gone well for both mother and baby. Then I introduced him to his new baby girl. He mouthed the word "Hope" and then said it out loud, his voice filled with pride. With the first glimpse of his daughter, he kept saying "she is so beautiful, so beautiful," and truly she was. C-Section babies usually miss the molded head and bruising that is often a part of the normal birthing process.

Mark followed me into the elevator to ride up to the nursery where civilization would begin to place its mark on Hope. Family members joined him to watch through the glass as we weighed, measured, and bathed her. I dressed Hope in a diaper and tee shirt than bundled her up in a fresh receiving blanket. As soon as Teresa arrived from recovery and had been settled in her room, I would take Hope to her for the bonding process to begin. Hope's entry into this world required emergency measures, and thankfully Teresa had chosen to deliver at a hospital where she could receive the care needed for Hope's safe arrival into this world.

Dr. Herman

• • •

Dr. Herman

• • •

THE CONTRAST BETWEEN BEING A student at the university medical hospital and working at this small community hospital, not 30 miles away, was never more graphically demonstrated than by the following strange experience.

Dr. Herman, I can't remember if Herman was his first or last name, but he was by far the oldest doctor delivering babies at our hospital, maybe *any* hospital. His patients were non-English speaking Mexican-American women who had heard through the grapevine that he had a kindly manner, and most importantly, that he and his wife (his office nurse) spoke Spanish.

Our department had a "cheat sheet" for translating a few appropriate words and phrases into Spanish. "Tierne dolor?" "Do you have pain?" Now, this one would seem pretty obvious as these women were often in advanced labor upon arrival. Culturally, and certainly in that era, women were very modest. Consequently, they chose to labor at home and waited until they *had* to come to the hospital.

None of these women had attended childbirth classes for a couple of good reasons. First, the classes were few and far between, and then were only offered in English. Naturally, by the time these expectant mothers came for admission, it was a bit late to teach the virtues of good breathing techniques. Even with our English-Spanish chart and a lot of gesturing, communications fell short often enough to frustrate staff and patients alike. The bewilderment on the women's faces made that clear.

Admitting instructions, left by each doctor, gave the nurses initial orders to provide care for their patients until they arrived. Dr. Herman had admitting instructions, too. His just didn't include anything for pain relief. He felt childbirth was a natural process, not one that needed any pain management *at all.*

Fortunately, for Dr. Herman's patients there were *unwritten* orders that the labor and delivery nurses all knew. The "procedure" involved calling his wife who would authorize pain medication. Dr. Herman never failed to co-sign her "verbal orders." I never understood the politics of that situation, but any questions I might have had seemed better left unasked.

Deliveries always seemed to catch Dr. Herman a little short of sleep, regardless of the time of day or night. In the delivery room he often started nodding off soon after making himself comfortable on the chrome wheeled, black leather stool. When his patient had a contraction and vocalized her discomfort, he opened his eyes briefly. Once the birth was imminent, meaning a dark-haired head crowning, the nurses made sure he was actually awake to deliver the newborn. It seemed like these catnaps went a bit beyond the intent of the "First do no harm" clause in the Hippocratic oath. Maybe it needed to start with "First be awake!"

So why did these patients come to Dr. Herman at all? I could only surmise that having a doctor who understood their language and culture carried a greater intrinsic value than any concern about his age, or his natural childbirth policy. Of course, his patients were unaware that Dr. Herman took naps in the delivery room while they labored. I do know his obstetric patients were treated with respect and dignity. Dr. and Mrs. Herman were gentle, kindhearted people who had served a Spanish-speaking population for many years as missionaries in Central America. They had moved to our small community to finish out their years of general practice before retirement, continuing to serve the Spanish-speaking population.

Jerri

• • •

Jerri

• • •

ON THE HOTTEST DAY I have ever experienced we moved our family from Santa Barbara to Golden Hills, a small town in Northern California. Soon after we were settled, I went to work part-time at the local 99-bed community hospital. By now, I had been out of school for twelve years. During this time I had gained experience: working in a doctor's office, teaching in the Regional Occupational Program (ROP), supervising home health aide's, and teaching nursing students at Santa Barbara City College. Even though I had come to this hospital with a variety of experiences, I soon found out there were many interesting challenges ahead.

I was working on the medical unit. One of the patients, Jerri, had an active gastro-intestinal (GI) bleed. She lay in the bed by the window, a nasal-gastric (NG) tube in her nose, draining blood-tinged secretions. Her face was pale, her lips chapped and pasty looking, consistent with her diagnosis of a stomach ulcer. Every two hours her NG tube was irrigated with ice-cold water in an attempt to cause the blood vessels and capillaries to contract, stopping the bleeding from her ulcer. With these treatments the membrane lining in the stomach *usually* heals rather rapidly.

When I went to her room to do the next irrigation, the gastric suction machine was draining *bright red* blood. I filled the 60 cc syringe with iced saline and worked as fast as I could, trying to get the fresh bleeding under control. Within minutes I realized the treatment wasn't slowing the flow of blood. I pulled the cord on the emergency light and asked the ward secretary to call for Jerri's doctor, STAT. If he did not respond immediately, another physician would be called in to manage Jerri's deteriorating condition.

Jerri was alert and well aware of her precarious situation. In a frail, frightened voice, she asked for a paper and pen to write a will, which seemed like a reasonable request that I relayed to the ward secretary. Her doctor's reputation with his peers was not stellar to say the least. He failed repeatedly to get needed second opinions or to make timely referrals to specialists on our hospital staff. Unfortunately, this time he was in the hospital.

Despite my STAT call, her doctor sauntered in, cowboy boots and all, and then just *stood* there. I told him the current IV was located in a small vein that would be inadequate for blood transfusions and it needed to be restarted. His response, given in his maddeningly, malaise voice was, "Oh, that won't be necessary. There's really nothing to get excited about here. I can handle everything." Ignoring him, I rushed out to get the IV tray with a supply of large gauge needles. Back at her bedside I proceeded to look for a new, larger vein. The timing was critical because the more blood she lost, the less likely it would be that I could get another IV line in. Under those circumstances a physician would need to place an Intercath in her subclavian vein. Who knew if this doctor had ever even *done* that procedure? I finally found a vein that was large enough and restarted her IV. Then I set it to run wide open to replace the lost volume in her circulatory system as quickly as possible until blood transfusions could be initiated.

Relieved with having a good IV line available, I turning to her doctor and asked "Are you going to contact a surgeon, or am I?" He muttered, almost inaudibly, that he would do it and grudgingly headed off towards the nurses' station. The ward clerk arrived with the paper and pen Jerri had requested. While she struggled to find a position to write her Will, I resumed the ice water irrigations, trying to keep us both calm as we waited anxiously for the surgeon to arrive.

Within minutes Dr. Sinclaire, our most respected surgeon arrived, sized up the situation, and called the OR staff to prepare for STAT surgery. Dr. Sinclaire controlled his temper enough not to say anything in front of the patient, but lit up with fury about the delayed referral out at the nurses' station, threatening never to take another referral from Jerri's doctor.

None of the nurses or medical staff members would blame Dr. Sinclaire if he lost Jerri during the surgery, but families aren't so forgiving. In their eyes the outcome would fall "in his court," regardless of the string of poor decisions made by Jerri's primary physician that created this life-threatening drama.

Jerri survived in spite of the almost-too-late surgical intervention. Since she was only in her early forties, she certainly deserved to be discharged home to her caring family, not taken out on a sheet-covered gurney to the local mortuary.

Not long after this incident, the Director of Nurses, Mr. Kragor, asked me if I wanted to apply for the position of Unit Manager on Station Four, a med-surg unit. I was interested, but hesitant, having heard horror stories about working for Mr. Kragor. He had a reputation for being an unhappy man who had no desire to see anyone else happy either. Stern and unbending were adjectives thrown about freely by the unit managers.

I decided to consult with the instructor for a Nurse Management class I had recently completed at the nearby university. I called her wanting her wisdom to help me make this decision. She graciously invited me to her house to discuss this opportunity to advance my nursing career in spite of the less-then-ideal superior. We sat outside on her patio looking down at her garden below and beyond to the green rolling hills, splashed with watercolor painted wild flowers. Wisely she advised me to consider accepting the position and to give my staff what I hoped to get from Mr. Kragor. Her perspective gave me the insight needed to join the nurse management team, a decision I have never regretted.

Ginger

• • •

Ginger

● ● ●

I HAD BEEN AT MY new position as Unit Manager for Station Four for several months. I enjoyed seeing my staff bloom under the positive rewards they were given for the unique contributions each made to the team. The recommendations my Nurse Management instructor had given me proved to be invaluable.

One day at the end of the shift, I started getting reports from my team to pass on to the next shift. The last came from one of my most conscientious nurses, giving her report on Ginger who had had a hysterectomy earlier in the day.

Ginger had been back from the recovery room for a couple of hours. When I had seen her on my rounds, the LVN was standing by her bed taking vital signs. Still groggy from surgery, Ginger's auburn curls lay tossed around her porcelain, oval-shaped face. Her husband sat at her bedside. As I walked by he bent down, brushed the curls from her forehead, and kissed her, a heart-warming picture.

Her orders called for the routine post-op vitals, observation of her surgical site dressing, and pain medication as needed. As I listened to the LVN giving a report on her vitals signs over the last hour, my ears perked up in concern. Ginger's last blood pressure was 70/40. This reading is low, *too low*. I asked to see Ginger's vital sign sheet. Her B/P had been dropping and her pulse rising consistently since her return from the recovery room. Both readings are signs of impending shock most likely from internal bleeding. This situation is critical, and the reason why patient's vital signs are so closely monitored after surgery.

I rushed to Ginger's room, set her IV to run wide open to, hopefully, keep her from going into shock, and then hurried back to the desk to call her surgeon with this disturbing report. He ordered a STAT blood count and asked me to call the OR staff, notifying them that Ginger would most likely be coming back for emergency surgery--just what I expected him to do.

The lab technician arrived within minutes. Ginger's nurse grabbed a gurney while I called for an orderly to assist in transporting Ginger. He would rush her up the elevator and then to the opposite corner of the hospital to the inconveniently located OR.

Grabbing Ginger's chart, I wrote the verbal orders and noted the actions taken. By then the surgeon had arrived to evaluate her. When the lab called with the report, I handed the phone to him. Her hemoglobin had dropped to 7.0 gms, precariously low, down from a pre-op level of 12.3 gms. His eyes widened as he ordered her back to surgery.

The orderly and LVN moved quickly to complete the pre-op checklist and to move her onto the gurney. I closed the chart to send with her and noticed the label on the front: NO BLOOD OR BLOOD DERIVATIVES in large red letters, taped across the front of her chart. My heart started pounding. Most likely she had a bleeder and without the option of blood transfusions, her prognosis would be greatly diminished. My heart sank.

We had sent her off to surgery that morning for an *elective* hysterectomy and now we were sending her back for *emergency* surgery, not knowing her chances of survival. With a great deal of reluctance, I called her husband with this worrisome update.

Feeling afraid that Ginger might not survive this second surgery, I wanted to scream at my nurse: "When were you going to get concerned about Ginger's vital signs?" Even if our patient had not elected to forgo blood transfusions, her vitals signs were still alarmingly low. Why had my LVN failed to see the significance of the vital signs she was monitoring? Had she forgotten what the word "vital" meant? Yes, she had taken the vitals as ordered, q 15 x 4 (every 15 minutes times four) and then q 30 x 2 (every 30 minutes times two) during the two hours Ginger had been back from the recovery room. She had been following orders to a "T," yet missing the whole point, jeopardizing our patient's life in the process.

I looked up to see Ginger's nurse's tear-streaked face. Devastation veiled her face as she now realized her part in creating this drama. Feeling compassion for her, I patted the chair beside me, indicating that she should sit down. What should I say to such a conscientious nurse about her error in judgment? Nothing. I knew she had already asked herself all the questions and that I no longer needed to. I asked her if she wanted to take an early lunch and she readily agreed, eager to get away from the atmosphere of our shaken unit. Now all we could do was wait to hear how Ginger weathered the next surgery.

Ginger's chances in the OR seemed slim at best. Our team got through the remainder of the shift, but left with heavy hearts. Later that evening I called ICU to see if she had survived the surgery. Ginger had, but they had found copious amounts of blood in her abdomen. She was hanging on by a thread. I felt no relief and slept very little that night. First thing in the morning I checked again. She had survived the night but just barely.

The next morning I wanted to stay home. Where had I failed in working with my team? Was my calm, optimistic personality setting my team up for feelings of complacence that could be life threatening? Was I naively confident in my staff? Had I not supervised them adequately? Would the Director of Nursing be waiting for me when I got to the hospital to relieve me of my position? Mr. Kragor was certainly not a "warm fuzzy" and was routinely *un*supportive of his staff, as well.

On the bright side: "Where there's life, there is hope." But my hope was hidden behind all these fears. I went in, of course. My staff would need support if Ginger didn't survive. We would need to do a "post-mortem" as a team to see how we had failed Ginger and most importantly, how we could prevent this from happening again.

The team was assembled in the report room when I arrived. Sober faces met my gaze and concern for Ginger's survival permeated the air. The night nurse was not particularly diplomatic, asking how we could have blown it so badly. What a start to the day.

Towards the end of the shift, I called the ICU again for an update. The surgeon said Ginger's chances of survival were now about 50/50, still not good. There had been only minimal response to the blood expanders (not blood derivatives) that she had been given, and her blood pressure and hemoglobin were still precariously low.

Her family had gathered in the ICU waiting room, vigilantly taking turns with the five-minute visits allowed. The pastor from their church had joined them for support. Ginger and her family were told repeatedly of the risk she was taking in not allowing blood transfusions, but she never wavered in her decision, a decision her family supported. Several more tense days passed for Ginger in ICU, but gradually she began showing signs of improvement. Toward the end of the week her condition stabilized and she was transferred back to our unit. A few days later she was discharged, going home to a very thankful family.

Everyone on our unit was very thankful as well, and now each team member had a much better idea of the meaning of taking *vital* signs!

"All Aboard"

• • •

"All Aboard"

● ● ●

WHEN NURSING HOME BEDS ARE scarce, discharge planners practically beg for beds, creating the opportunity for nursing home operators to be choosy. Naturally patients who can afford to pay cash get first priority. Patients on public assistance have the longest waits, particularly if they require much in the way of nursing care. We often had one or two of these patients waiting on our unit.

These marginalized patients need to be viewed as individuals of dignity and worth. Some had interesting life stories they could share with us. Other patient's stories were locked in minds clouded by various stages of senility. Families filled us in on the life of these patients and brought pictures from younger years, before time and gravity had had its way with their features. Memorabilia, hung on corkboards above their beds, helped us gain respect and an understanding of the lives these patients had led.

One patient, Henry, seemed to be the last leaf on his family tree. When he came to our unit, we asked questions about his life history. He didn't share much with us other than the fact that he had spent his life as an engineer on railways, criss-crossing the United States. His wife had passed away years before. They had no children. Henry, at eighty-seven, seemed strangely resigned to his solitary station in life and to his deteriorating condition. No visitor broke the monotony for him. We did our best to visit with him when other responsibilities allowed. His nurses often left his TV on, tuned to a nature or history channel to fill up the empty spaces in his room. We soon found that Henry didn't respond well to having other patients in his room, seeming to prefer his own company. As often as possible, we left the other bed empty.

As he waited for a nursing home bed, he became progressively more debilitated. Eventually he lapsed into a semi-comatose state with fewer and fewer moments of lucidity. We knew Henry's time was short and that he might pass away before his transfer. By then, our staff began to hope discharge planning *wouldn't* find a bed for him. It didn't seem right for strangers to care for him in his final days.

One day as I passed his room, I noticed a program about steam trains on his TV screen. Henry's eyes were open and he was more alert than we had seen him in days. I went to get my assistant RN to show her this strange "awakening." When we got to Henry's room he was still lucid, even pointing a gnarled finger at the screen. He didn't have the strength to talk, so we commented about *his* days as an engineer with the railway, giving *him* recognition for the life he lived and the service *he* had provided to so many travelers. A brief smile crossed his face as he sank back into the pillow, eyes closing. We watched transfixed as Henry's final breaths left his body, a treasured memory of a good passing for a tired old engineer taking his final train ride.

Mushrooms to Die For

● ● ●

Mushrooms to Die For

• • •

MUSHROOMS HAVE NEVER COME CLOSE to being on *my* grocery list. I know other people eat mushrooms, even like them. I just couldn't understand why anyone would go *looking* for them in the forest. Consequently, when we admitted three young "kids" in their early 20's for mushroom poisoning, I though, "Why didn't they just buy the mushrooms? Why risk misidentifying them?" This experience came before I had met anyone with a "hippy" background who could fill me in on life outside my little bubble.

The three young adults, two males and a female, had arrived code three at our emergency room with violent episodes of vomiting and diarrhea. On admission, samples of the mushrooms were sent for identification and the Poison Control Center had been called. Treatment in the ER included pumping their stomachs (even though nature was making a valiant effort to rid their bodies of the toxins on its own) and the administration of IV fluids with the electrolytes needed to replace what they had already lost and were continuing to lose. At that point, the three were transferred to our unit.

Unfortunately, what they were trying to find in the forest and what they actually got were two entirely different things. They were looking for mushrooms that would provide them with a psychedelic high, but had gotten much more than they bargained for. Ingestion of the type of poisonous wild mushroom they had stumbled upon was literally a death sentence in the days before liver transplants.

When their doctor told me the dire prognosis, her words felt like rocks hitting my chest, only to lodge in my stomach. It seemed hypocritical to be going into their room with medications that I now knew would only ease their gastro-intestinal symptoms. It felt like taking band-aides to someone hemorrhaging from gunshot wounds. What could I say to them? They hadn't heard their prognosis yet. How could I sound encouraging? How could I look any one of them in the eye? At this point they looked healthy enough, a little "green around the gills" perhaps, but not at death's door.

This trio had Dr. Ella, a young female doctor, handling their care. What a frustrating situation for her. The deadly poison they had ingested was tying her hands. Every cell in her body must have wanted to undo the damage they had done. In the time it took them to hike out of the forest and be transported by ambulance to our hospital, the toxins had already wreaked havoc within their bodies. Soon after these patients reached our unit, Dr. Ella contacted a University Hospital in San Francisco to discuss transferring them there for definitive care.

Before their families arrived at our hospital, the trio was on their way to San Francisco. After the sound of the helicopters faded into the distance, Dr. Ella told us the transfers had been done primarily to make sure everything possible would be done to save these young lives, even though chances of survival for them were slim.

The specialist at the teaching hospital would put them on dialysis, but had offered little hope for their survival. Several days later we got the news that the two young men had succumbed to the poison. Then the following day the young woman lost her battle. They paid a heavy price for their youthful indiscretion. The tragic outcome we more or less expected left a sense of futility and loss in its wake.

"Just Hurry"

• • •

"Just Hurry"

● ● ●

THE QUIET OF OUR UNIT evaporated the moment the elevator opened and
Dr. Jensen stepped out, desperately trying to hold on to a convulsing baby.
She had come directly from her office next door. I raced to help her with
the baby as Billi, my LVN, grabbed a crib and shoved it into the procedure
room.

Dr. Jensen's practice was primarily for well-baby checkups, treatment
of "bumps and bruises" along with the typical illnesses of childhood, so it
was rare for her to admit *any* of her patients to the hospital. Most often, she
referred the "sicker" babies and children to the two other pediatricians on
staff for hospital management.

She was shrieking verbal orders as she handed me the seizing baby to
swaddle. First, Dr. Jensen ordered a STAT dose of Valium to be given IV
to stop the seizures. However, Dr. Jensen didn't start her own IV's as the
other two pediatricians did. Our unit had two nurses (one off duty, the
other at lunch) who were certified to start IV's on infants, but I hadn't
been certified yet. Dr. Jensen's voice came tumbling out high and tight as
she yelled the obvious. "We've got to stop these seizures *now*! She's been
convulsing for several minutes! Get that IV started now!" Billi had anticipated this and had IV supplies and the Valium ready. The only missing
piece was someone qualified to start the IV. I just wanted to disappear!

Yes, I had observed this procedure performed by others many times,
but *observing* is a far cry from doing. My mind raced to find an alter-
nate plan. None emerged. This needed to be done *now*. Even with Billi

restraining the baby, she was still a moving target. With a shaky heart and as steady a hand as I could muster, I miraculously placed the "butterfly" needle into a tiny vein on her scalp, while listening to Dr. Jensen anxiously repeating, "Just hurry, just hurry, get the Valium in." Billi drew up the Valium, which we checked together (with the "just hurry's" still filling the room) before I administered it. Within seconds, the baby's little body began to relax. Lucky baby. It took *my* body the rest of the day!

Roger's Angst

• • •

Roger's Angst

● ● ●

*(The American Journal of Nursing published
a version of this story in April 2011)*

HE WAS STANDING IN OUR small utility room, under florescent lights, hands on the counter, head down. Instinctively, I started quietly backing out, thinking he wanted privacy. "Don't go," he said in a low, gravelly voice. He shook his head slowly in disbelief: "I have to give up nursing." Seconds ticked by as I wondered what could possibly be so serious to prompt such a *drastic* decision? Did he have cancer? AIDS?

Roger was older than many on our floor, his coal black hair woven with gray, a quiet, competent leader with over 10 years of experience at our hospital. He had served as a medic in the Gulf Wars. He was conscientious about his responsibilities to his team members and patients. His performance reviews were excellent. As the head nurse on the afternoon shift, he'd arrive early to organize his duties. His staff appreciated his calming influence during the sometimes frantic pace of our med-surg unit.

At last it came out, "I almost hung the wrong blood on my patient!" The words dropped like a curtain, leaving him with his thoughts, me with mine. I eased the door closed with my foot, mentally reviewing policies and procedures, looking for answers to the "how" and "why."

"But you didn't," I told him. A platitude too quickly spoken. Roger's response was full of self-loathing, "But I could have!" After a few moments he sighed and continued, saying he had taken the lab slip to the blood bank, found the unit with her name on it, but somehow, grabbed the *wrong* one. He hadn't discovered his error until he checked his patient's name band. "I could have *killed* my patient," Roger said, his voice still thick with pent-up anger.

"Yes, but *you* caught your error," I said. "The blood administration protocol worked!" No response. "There'd be no need for those last two checks if nurses were robots, but *we* aren't." He didn't respond, so I pushed on. I told him that if he were the only medical professional to *ever* make an error, then yes, he should quit, but he had to be aware of errors others had made. At this, he nodded slightly.

"You're an integral part of this unit," I said. "We need *you*, our patients need *your* expertise, *your* compassion." I fell silent. At last he looked up at me through moist eyes and nodded. My cue to leave.

After the shift report, Roger came to me and requested the next day off as a "mental health day." I noticed that he had the following two days off as well. I hoped that during this time he'd regain some balance.

On the way out to my car, I stopped in the cafeteria for a cup of tea. I found a table in a corner where I could decompress from the shift. However serious his error had almost been, Roger's conclusion to *quit* nursing seemed utterly irrational. Trying to help him gain perspective had left me drained.

Then an experience of mine came rushing back in full color. Early in my career I'd taken a position at a new hospital. I wanted to make a good impression. Instead, I made a serious medication error. I remember the terror I felt, the mixture of shame and fear as I filled out the incident report, and headed home to a sleepless night. In our thin-walled condo, our master bedroom backed up to the utility room of our neighbor, a high school PE teacher. Every night we went to bed hearing his tennis shoes bounce around the dryer as an unwelcome lullaby. This night the rhythmic sound seemed to be saying accusingly, "How could you?" "How could you?" "How *could* you!" I lay there, silently crying, feeling the weight of the shame--so ashamed I didn't even tell my husband--denying myself the comfort he would have willingly given me.

The next day, as I prepared my medication tray with shaking hands, two physicians sat at the nurses' station, talking loudly as they discussed *the* medication error, wondering which nurse had made it. Overhearing them, I turned and confessed, feeling like a marked woman. They muttered something in my direction, shook their heads, and quickly returned to their charting.

For weeks afterwards I expected to be terminated. For years I told no one about my shameful experience. My "little secret" occasionally popped up in my mind, bringing tightness to my chest, eating away at my confidence. Later, when teaching nursing students to pass medications, I didn't use my own medication error as an example, my perfectionism wouldn't allow it.

As my tea grew tepid, I began to understand why Roger's response--and my own, for all those years--seemed out of proportion to the crime. They were. Roger's expectation of personal perfection had blurred the mirror he used to evaluate himself as a nurse. What do we, as conscientious nurses need when we make a mistake? I believe we need time to evaluate the situation, to learn from it—and then we need the healing salve of compassion from those who stand beside us and those who lead us.

On the fourth day Roger returned. When he walked out of the elevator with his head held high and his back straight, I felt certain that the time off had been beneficial. He came over to see me at the nurses' desk. This time when our eyes met he said, with a smart salute and a smile playing around his eyes, "Roger, Registered Nurse, reporting for duty." Roger *had* forgiven himself. I could not have been more pleased. Roger had weathered the storm.

Mrs. Jones

● ● ●

Mrs. Jones

• • •

MRS. JONES HAD BEEN ADMITTED with a fractured hip from a nasty spill she had taken at home. In her late seventies, she had been living alone for the last few years after the death of her husband. Her bright, optimistic and appreciative attitude made her a delight to have as a patient. She had an aura of refinement surrounding her--we were not even *tempted* to address her by her given name. Her three sons, all attorneys, lived in the area. It was evident that they cared a great deal about their mother's well being, and at least one of them came to visit her each evening.

The private room she had been given was alive with many arrangements of fresh flowers. Their fragrance, intertwined with her own perfume, made it a sensory pleasure to enter her room. In deference to her station in life, my most sophisticated nurses provided care for her. As Head Nurse on my unit I made rounds at least twice a day on all my patients, but I have to confess, I often spent more time in Mrs. Jones' room than her condition warranted just to savor the ambiance.

Several days after surgery, Mrs. Jones decided she wanted a shower. After all, her room came with a private bathroom with a shower. The doctor's current orders read: bed rest and bathroom privileges, but only with assistance. "Would you kindly call my doctor to see if he might change my order to include a shower?" She asked this with her normal easy tone and sweet smile. It didn't seem like an unreasonable request to her. "After all, the physical therapist who has been working with me said that I am doing exceptionally well with my walker." Now she proudly used the walker for trips to "the powder room," as her nurse stood by.

I felt caught between Mrs. Jones request, a slight feeling of hesitancy, and a doctor who generally agreed with my requests for changes in his treatment plan. Finally, I agreed to call him, and not surprisingly, he gave an order for her desired shower. Her bedside nurse was happy to be able to please her with this seemingly benign request.

Soon the steam filled her bathroom and billowed out into her room. I stopped by to see her, probably hoping to hear appreciation for getting her order changed. When I got there, Mrs. Jones was up, using her walker with her nurse at her side, heading for the bathroom and her beloved shower. It felt good to see her up and so pleased with herself.

Not five minutes later the light above Mrs. Jones' door flashed *red*, meaning assistance was needed immediately. Several of us arrived almost at the same time and most unfortunately, found Mrs. Jones lying on the floor of the shower moaning in pain. I couldn't believe my eyes! Why hadn't I just said "No" to her request? A small part of me *had* felt reluctant to call her doctor. Why hadn't I listened?

With more than enough help to get her onto a gurney, I went to make the dreaded call to her doctor. On the way I stopped off in the small kitchenette near her room. Two nurses were in there agonizing over this latest turn of events. The first word out of my mouth was *"Damn,"* a word the staff had never heard me utter. They stood there shocked, then began to giggle at my embarrassment that such a word had slipped out. But what else is there to say when your first thoughts hadn't been about Mrs. Jones but were about those three doting sons of hers who all happened to be attorneys? I feared my job could be in jeopardy and I was upset that a favorite patient had to go through the pain and disability from a second surgery--one that I felt responsible for. Why had I made that call?

Necessary arrangements were made. The X-ray technician arrived promptly to take the portable films and soon Mrs. Jones was on her way back to OR for a *second* repair of her fractured hip. The incident reports were filled out and the Director of Nurses was notified. (He was never a "happy camper," and this certainly would bring a barrage of accusatory words.) Why had I accepted this position as Head Nurse anyway?

When she was fully alert and oriented in the Recovery Room, Mrs. Jones was returned to her room. All three of her distressed sons were waiting for her there. The most composed person throughout this unfortunate turn of events was Mrs. Jones herself. To their credit, "the boys," as she called them, listened to their mother when she told them her story. She confessed that she had *insisted* the doctor be called because she could not go *one* more day without a shower. Then she added that there would be "no fuss" (meaning legal action) about this *little* setback. To my great amazement, there was none. I learned from this experience not to be beguiled by sweet, sophisticated ladies of any age!

Thanksgiving Day

● ● ●

Thanksgiving Day

● ● ●

ON THANKSGIVING DAY I WAS scheduled to be the Relief House Supervisor for the day shift. Having only done this twice, I felt the Director of Nurses' trust in my ability to handle this responsibility was ill founded. Having agreed to do it, I faced the day with trepidation. My concern was my limited experience along with the Thanksgiving Day holiday that is traditionally the busiest of the year. What if a rash of accidents filled the ER to overflowing? These two factors alone could test my ability as a Relief Supervisor, and who knew what other challenges I would need to face? But whatever the shift might throw at me, I could look forward to my flight to Santa Barbara later that afternoon for Thanksgiving Dinner with my family.

For the first couple of hours, the shift was basically quiet. As I made my rounds I noted that the ICU was well staffed, a blessing I might need if the ER called for extra help. This eased my anxiety, but just a little. Around mid-day my beeper went off, startling me. Would I ever feel comfortable with that sound? I didn't know. The call was from the ER. They had a sudden increase in census.

One of their cases, a four-year-old named Cindy, had arrived with symptoms of epiglottis (a swelling of the throat) that threatened to asphyxiate her. This condition, a complication of the flu, though rare, is often fatal. I paged ICU, telling them I needed an extra nurse STAT in ER. Richard, the nurse from ICU, and I arrived almost simultaneously. Richard immediately joined the circle of bright lights illuminating the team working on Cindy. I stayed, absorbing the electric energy in the room, knowing an extra hand might be needed to help. Jane, the hospital's social worker stood with the parents, encouraging them to go with her to the Quiet Room. The father refused vehemently as his wife silently sobbed into his chest. Cindy's mother cannot watch and her father cannot leave as his instinctual role of protector keeps him there. I could have paged security to escort them out of the ER, but what right did I have? Would it be for my own comfort to have the family "safely" tucked away somewhere? Cindy's parents were not interfering as they stayed in support of a daughter unaware of their presence.

Dr. Baker, a general practitioner, headed the team working feverishly over the child, yet her condition continued to deteriorate. Soon CPR was initiated and continued for almost an hour. Her doctor quietly canceled it and noted the time of death as 12:59 p.m. It seemed the air had been sucked out of the room by the loss of Cindy's little life. Emergency Room staff members listlessly gathered up the remains of a failed effort. No one spoke. Silence prevailed.

Dr. Baker's halting steps indicated his reluctance to meet with Cindy's family. Yet, this is part of his role as a physician and a most difficult one. Eventually he joined the social worker standing with the parents to explain. To explain what? Explain that everything that was done for Cindy still didn't save her life. I question whether they would believe him. I'm not sure I believed him? Cindy's parents were allowed and encouraged to spend time with their daughter, at her bedside, the first step in their grieving process. Sounds of sobbing swirled around the room as I slipped silently through the swinging doors. Back at the supervisor's office I closed the door and slumped, exhausted, into the swivel chair.

There my thoughts returned to Cindy's case. Why had her tragic death happened? Should a pediatrician have been called in? Should she have been airlifted to a larger hospital? My mind kept trying to fix the unfixable as my heart continued to ache for Cindy's family. My mind wondered if Thanksgiving would ever be the same for them, although my heart knew it would not. Eventually this dreadful shift ended and I headed wearily and without focus to my car and then to the airport.

On the flight down to be with my family, I realized I needed to turn my thoughts to life outside the hospital. Our Thanksgiving dinner ought to be a time to reflect on the blessings of the past year, a time to realize how fortunate we are to live in "the land of the free," and just to be alive at all. I needed to stow away the pain over the loss of Cindy, but how? My mind wandered to other professionals who are faced with similar tragedies of life: Highway Patrol Officers, Fire and Police personnel, Search and Rescue teams and, of course, our Armed Forces. Thank God for those who are willing to deal with life at its worst, helping to create a safer world for us to enjoy. I looked forward to being enfolded in the love of my family, even though they would not know how desperately I needed it. I would bask in the comfort of their arms.

The following week I made an appointment to meet with Dr. Baker at his modest office in a small complex behind the hospital to discuss the four-year-old girl we had lost on Thanksgiving Day. A knot in my stomach developed as I sat in his waiting room, wondering if I would be able to hold my emotions in check as I talked to him. Part of my mission would be to seek reassurance that our staff had done their very best to save Cindy.

And yet, the greater unasked question would be, "Had *he* missed anything?" I knew he had seen Cindy in his office the day before she died. Should he have done things differently at that time? As we sat in his small, cluttered office, I noticed family pictures mixed in with medical artifacts among the crowded bookshelves behind his desk. He greeted me as he pulled up a chair for me. Our conversation started out stilted. "How was your Thanksgiving?" "Fine, we got back yesterday. How was yours?" Etc. Eventually I was able to bring the conversation around to Cindy. Talking with him about the progression of her illness gave me some relief. Hearing more about her initial symptoms, his examination and treatment plan on the day prior to Thanksgiving helped me begin to accept the unacceptable. I heard fatigue in his voice, saw strain etched in his face, and sensed the loss he felt. Finally our conversation melted into a reflective silence.

As I stood to leave, Dr. Baker came from behind his desk and put an arm around my shoulder, giving it a gentle squeeze of support. The moments passed with both of us seemingly unable to say good-bye. In the end our silence said what we could not. Turning to leave, I gave him a weak smile, hoping he would see my "Thank you" behind it. The loss of Cindy lay just a little lighter on my heart because of our shared time of reflection. How could I not come away with greater respect for Dr. Baker as a person and physician?

Sometimes, everything you do is still not enough and you are left with shattered lives and broken dreams. Regardless of your level of education, area of expertise, or the institution you are working for, the fight for life is sometimes lost. People die. Naturally, it is that much harder when it is a child. Yet, you have to show up the next day and try again to comfort the dying and care for the living. As a team you will provide support to one another so you can each go about your duties. That is the often un-discussed, yet, the reality of the medical field.

Baby Michael's Story

• • •

Baby Michael's Story

• • •

I TURNED THE CORNER TO our unit one January morning, a few minutes before the start of the morning shift. The sky, cold and grey, hung low overhead. It had looked the same—day after day after day. Come to think of it, I'm not sure when we had last seen the sun. Our small town sat on the edge of the foothills of the Sierra Nevada's. Unfortunately, we were just not high enough above the central valley floor to keep us above the dampening fog of winter. Here we were, just a few weeks past Christmas and most of the staff, including myself, had at least a touch of the post-holiday blues.

Station Four was primarily a Med-Surg unit, yet frequently we also cared for infants and children, making the mix more interesting and challenging. A crib in the hall alerted me that the patient census was high. The large crib dwarfed the tiny infant inside. Even from a distance, the hollows around the baby's eyes were haunting. Two IV's were hanging, their monitors beeping, punctuating the medley of early morning sounds as the day shift rituals began.

The phlebotomist had arrived for early morning blood draws. Surgical patients had been awakened for final pre-op routines. Early bird doctors were drinking coffee and chatting with the night nurses. An aide was emptying catheter bags to complete the Intake and Output records for the night shift; others were sitting at the chart racks recording final notes. Patients, awakened from sleep by pain, were anxiously awaiting the sound of the medication nurses' shoes softly padding down the hall.

The day shift would soon be taking vital signs and handing a wet washcloth (hopefully warm) to the patients for a.m. care. If time permitted, some patients might even get oral care prior to breakfast. Next would come the clatter of the breakfast cart being wheeled off the elevator, awakening any patients who had somehow managed to sleep through these early morning activities.

In the midst of this cacophony, the baby slept, bunched up, unaware of the activities swirling around. I hoped the baby was just a sound sleeper and not too sick to respond to all the noise and commotion.

My first responsibility would be making staff assignments. The "wisp of life" in the hall would be assigned to Billi, an LVN. She had a special touch with babies. The smaller they were, the better she liked caring for them, and in emergency situations she stayed calm and efficient. This baby looked like it just might need her special skills before the end of our shift.

Even though I also love babies, I decided to keep myself busy with other things and to keep my distance from the crib as much as possible. "Pick your battles" translates to "pick your emotional pains" in the health care arena. Walls around my emotions were already being erected and hopefully they would shield me from this potential loss.

Billi stood almost six feet tall, with a full, sturdy figure. Short blond curls framed her round, pleasant face. A guess at her age would put her in her mid-thirties, not that much younger than I, yet our backgrounds were worlds apart. While I came from a sheltered childhood, lived in middle class communities, and attended private Christian schools for my entire education, Billi had grown up in this rural community and attended local schools that were full of drugs and were notoriously sub-standard academically. Yet, amazingly Billi had gone to the local Junior College and completed her LVN degree. I had a sense that she had seen a lot of life in her years, the kind of life that makes for good lyrics in country western songs. I liked her earthiness. Billi came with no pretense; she stood behind no mask. What you saw was what you got. She knew herself, and seemed comfortable in her own skin.

One day Billi's size, strength, and edgy background proved to be more than two tough teen-age boys expected. The two had crossed paths and traded punches outside a "shared" girlfriend's hospital room. Billi grabbed both of them by the scruffs of their necks and tossed them out the back door before they had a clue of what had happened.

Today, she came to shift report with her engaging smile and positive attitude. We would need that ray of sunshine. The night nurse's report on the seven-week old infant in the hall wasn't encouraging. He had been admitted to our floor from the emergency room in the early morning hours. His diagnoses included: Failure to Thrive, Bilateral Pneumonia, a ruptured eardrum, dehydration and, if that wasn't enough, a badly excoriated bottom. Even the experience I had received on the Pediatric Unit at the University Hospital had not prepared me for this. This baby looked like he had been taking care of himself and hadn't been doing a very good job of it. "By the way," I asked quizzically, "where is his mother?" A question that would soon become rhetorical. The night nurse responded that she left within minutes of his admission and hadn't been seen since. Strange.

He weighed less than five pounds, down from a birth weight of over seven. Not good. His lab work and spinal tap to rule out meningitis had been done. His spinal fluid and blood samples had been sent to the lab for STAT analysis. His blood work showed a high white count, confirming that his little body had a serious infection. Blood cultures had been done, but the results would take at least 24 hours before the bacteria could be identified and a specific antibiotic ordered. In his favor, the report on his spinal fluid came back clear, ruling out meningitis.

He had arrived from ER with IV fluids to re-hydrate him and two IV antibiotics. The pediatrician hoped that one of them would attack the bacteria that had invaded his tiny body. His name was Michael, making him more than a number. All of this was more than I wanted to hear.

Not long after the shift report was over, Dr. Carrington, a pediatrician on staff, the one I had the most confidence in, came to examine Michael and to get a detailed history from his family. He looked shocked, his brow furrowed, his eyes wide open, when he heard that Michael's mother had left almost immediately after his admission, hours before, and had not been seen since. Dr. Carrington asked me to try to contact her. I grabbed his chart and flipped to the admission sheet and found his mother's name, Sally Hedges. No home phone number was listed for her, just a number where a message could be left. I picked up the receiver and dialed the number. No answer and no message machine. Dr. Carrington asked me to keep trying to reach her and to have her call his office ASAP (as soon as possible).

8:30 a.m. T.C. (telephone call) to Sally's message number. No answer. EL /RN

By eleven o'clock I was on edge. Michael's mother had not shown up. Usually parents hover around the hospital, often around the clock, trying to catch "cat naps" in the reclining chairs provided for them, anxious to get updates as soon as they were available. Naturally, they were also there to provide love and support for their sick baby or child.

Just before going to lunch, I redialed the message number listed for Sally. A gruff sounding male voice answered the phone. "No she's not here. No! I don't know when I'll see her and don't call so early again!" Then I asked him his name. "My name? You have *got* to be kidding," and then followed the sharp click of the receiver being slammed down in my ear.

"Eleven o'clock, early? Really?" This thought crossed my (occasionally judgmental) mind as I took Michael's chart out of the rack to record this conversation.

11:00 a.m. T.C. to message phone for mother. Uncooperative male unhelpful with whereabouts of Sally Hedges. EL/RN

By the end of the day shift, Billi's report on Michael was brief. There had been no signs of improvement, but he had held his own. Then she added that Michael must be "a tough little guy" to have survived the shift. It had been difficult for me to avoid his crib as I tried valiantly not to see what I did not want to know. It would be harder yet to go home, without taking at least a part of him with me in my heart.

3:00 p.m. T.C. Another attempt to reach Michael's mother w/o success. Dr. Carrington notified. He requested that the p.m. shift continue trying to reach her. EL/RN

Cold whipping wind and drippy fog met me as I scurried to my car, relieved that the emotionally draining shift had finally ended. Despite the inclement weather, I went shopping, more to distract myself than out of need. At home, the family rituals of cooking dinner, cleaning the kitchen, helping the kids with homework, and finally tucking them into bed were exactly what I needed to keep my mind off of Michael. Exhausted, I fell into bed, but visions of Michael's tiny, emaciated body interrupted my sleep, leaving me un-rested when the alarm insisted another day had arrived.

The next morning when I arrived on my unit, I noticed that Michael's crib was still in the hall. He had not slipped away in the night. Michael lay huddled and bundled, now with one of the IV's placed in his head. The night shift reported that his temperature had remained high, fluctuating little through the night. One of his IV's had infiltrated and had been restarted; otherwise, there had been no change. Still his mother had not come!

As assignments were being made, I asked Billi if she needed a break from Michael. She shook her head and said "No way!" I felt a sense of relief, knowing he could be in no better hands. Like a surrogate mother she would spend as much time as possible by his crib, talking to him, touching him, willing him to live.

Dr. Carrington arrived early to examine Michael. Concern clouded his face when he heard that Michael's mother *still* hadn't been in to see him. He grabbed the phone, flipped open the chart to get the number and dialed. With no answer, his balled fist hit the desk as he hung up asking the unanswerable question: "Where is that woman?" His tone, words and facial expression adamantly conveyed that Sally no longer fit his description of a mother. She didn't fit ours either. A very small part of me wondered if she might be in a coma at some other hospital. I didn't want to accept that she had abandoned Michael. Mothers just don't do that! As Dr. Carrington stood to leave, he asked me to have the nursing staff keep trying to contact her. I reached for the Nursing Care Plan and added in bold writing:

> *Try to reach Michael's mother at least twice during the a.m. and p.m. shifts.*

Eventually, the Social Service Department would have to be notified if Sally didn't respond to our messages.

> *3:00 p.m. T.C. Unable to reach Michael's mother per phone after several attempts during the shift. A man answered and reluctantly agreed to pass a message along "If and when he saw Sally." Dr. Carrington's office and Social Services (S.S.) notified. EL/RN*

Thankfully, I had the next two days off. I felt emotionally drained and hoped to come back feeling recharged. When back at the hospital, I turned the corner to our unit and instantly noticed Michael's crib was missing from the hall. My heart dropped, but a quick look at the census reassured me that he was still here. He had just been moved to Room 403, directly across the hall from our nurses' station, thank God. This time the night shift's report gave some better news. Michael's temperature had come down significantly and the congestion in his lungs had begun to clear.

When I came out of the nurse's report room, I found Dr. Carrington sitting at the nurses' desk, writing a progress note on Michael. He was pleased with his progress, but even more frustrated and concerned that there had been no contact from his "mother." To pursue the cause of Michael's Failure to Thrive, the doctor needed to know what formula Michael's mother had given him, if she had breast fed him, and most importantly, how he had handled those feedings. Differential diagnoses included: an intolerance of milk based formula, a digestive system too immature to absorb feedings, pyloric stenosis (narrowing of the outlet of the stomach, allowing very little of his feedings to pass into his intestines) causing projectile vomiting and weight loss. If Michael had pyloric stenosis, he would soon need surgical intervention. Then there remained the *remote* possibility that Michael had not been fed adequate amounts. Unfortunately, we had no clues since Sally Hedges had *still* not returned our calls or come to see her baby.

Dr. Carrington had no choice but to pursue Michael's Failure to Thrive without his "mother's" input. He started by ordering bottle-feeding of sterile water using a preemie nipple, making it easy for Michael to suck. He would continue receiving IV fluids until his oral intake was adequate.

Michael tried a bit of the sterile water during his first feeding but only took an ounce. Fortunately his nurse noticed no difficulty in swallowing or retaining it. Soon Michael progressed to glucose water. Michael had no vomiting, colic or apparent problems with his digestion. With that information, the next day Dr. Carrington ordered a trial of diluted milk-based formula. Once again there were no signs of problems, so Michael was advanced to full strength formula the following day. By now he would take at least three ounces before falling back to sleep.

Over the next week Michael began gaining back the weight he had lost since birth. The weight loss problem didn't seem to be a Failure to Thrive issue, but a failure to *feed*! With this suspicion of neglect, Dr. Carrington notified Child Protective Services (CPS) as required by law and asked me to give an update to the hospital's Social Service Department.

3:00 p.m. T.C. to the Social Services re: Michael's status, Dr. Carrington's suspicions of neglect, and our numerous unsuccessful attempts to reach his mother, Sally Hedges. Social Services will open a case on Michael and try to reach his mother as well. EL/RN

Several days later the night shift reported that Michael's mother *had* finally come in around 1:30 a.m. Sally identified herself at the desk, and the team leader told her Dr. Carrington had been trying to reach her for almost a week about Michael. He needed to hear from her ASAP! She just gave a half-hearted shrug and entered Michael's room. The team leader followed her and stood by the door. Sally stayed for less than five minutes and left without even touching or holding Michael. The RN repeated the urgent need for her to contact the doctor. She snapped, "I heard you the first time," and continued in a huff down the hall towards the elevator.

Now that Michael's infections had cleared up and he was on oral feedings, Sara, my ward secretary, and I got a bassinet and brought him behind the nurses' desk, more for our benefit than his, I'm sure. Because of our love of babies, it seemed the natural thing to do. Now, Michael needed to gain a sufficient amount of weight to be ready for discharge, *but to whom?* Surely not to his elusive "mother." We were all concerned about Michael's future. Michael, so tiny, so vulnerable, and so absolutely adorable, had wormed his way into our hearts. He even had "fans" from other areas of the hospital who looked for reasons to come by and see him. Soon he began rewarding us with smiles that showed off his dimples.

Sara, in her late twenties, was short, with curves, and had wavy sandy-blonde hair that fell just above her shoulders. Highly efficient, she had a pleasing personality, making coming to work a pleasure. Her gregarious personality was made complete by a laugh that bubbled up often (but never inappropriately), helping to keep stress levels in check. It takes a finely tuned awareness of what is happening on the unit at any given time to keep the wheels turning. Sara had these gifts. She had good interpersonal skills with the physicians, didn't let their occasional grumblings upset her, and she could even *read* the "chicken scratch" they often left as orders.

Sara and her husband, Bob, had been trying to have a baby for several years. One day she was feeding Michael when she blurted out that she and her husband had been talking about adopting the night before. She looked down into Michael's big eyes that were now turning blue, and commented wistfully, "It just seems so unfair that Michael's mother got pregnant and she doesn't even care enough to come see him!" Her voice trailed off into silence. I could say nothing to make it better, her plaintive words cutting at my heart.

Still in a musing mode, I turned to Sara and said, "If Michael's mother stopped by right now, we could tell her there was a couple that would love to provide a home for Michael. And then casually mention that they would be willing to reimburse her, just like one would with a surrogate mother." Michael started to cry, bringing our reverie to an end. Sara hoisted him up over her shoulder to burp him, gently patting and massaging his tiny back. When he nodded off to sleep, she tucked him back into his bassinet. We knew my musing was in vain. Feelings of frustration over Michael's situation hung between us once more.

Because of Sally Hedge's absence from Michael's life during the two weeks since his admission, Social Services had written a standing order on the chart to contact their department immediately if *anyone* came to see him. One day an aunt, his father's sister, came to visit. Billi was bathing Michael when she arrived. Trailing behind the aunt came a toddling little girl, shyly cute with sun-streaked sandy hair, and trailing behind her, a raggedy blanket. The aunt, who called herself Betty Jo, picked up the little girl and caught Billi totally off guard by saying, "You know, this here is Michael's sister, Megan. I think Sally said they were like fifteen months apart." Finally, a connection with *someone* in Michael's family! Later, Billi told me she had to bite her lip to stay calm after Betty Jo dropped this bombshell.

The woman and the toddler had caught my eye as they passed the desk and headed, without stopping, to Michael's room. I immediately notified our Social Service Department. The Social Worker that answered sounded frazzled, saying she couldn't come right now, as she was busy with another patient's family. "Could you ask her to stay around for a few minutes? I know how important this contact is for Michael. I will come just as soon as possible!" Raising my eyebrows, I replaced the receiver and hoped that would be soon enough. Then I slipped down to the door to Michael's room, hoping to eavesdrop on the conversation, hoping to delay her, and looking for answers to the often-repeated question, "Where is Michael's mother?"

Billi continued an easy conversation with Betty Jo as she gave Michael his bath. As she was finishing, she asked Betty Jo to hand her the towel. Betty Jo couldn't get over how much weight he had gained, and how healthy he looked. Billi agreed saying, "If Michael continues gaining like this he'll be ready to go home soon. Oh! I'd better get a diaper on this little guy quick before he pees all over me!" which got both of them giggling. Then Billi went on to say, "The only thing Dr. Carrington needs to do before he can discharge Michael is to talk to his mother in person."

When Billi asked if Betty Jo would pass that message along to Sally, she gave a shrug in frustration, saying "Sure, next time I see her, and who knows when the hell that'll be? She's been hit'n the bottle so much worse since she and Michael's father got back together again. I've had this little one here," nodding at Megan, "for well over a month. Sally hardly comes to see her and won't even take Megan home with her to give me a break, even for a little while." Pausing to sigh and catch her breath, she stammered in frustration "wherever *home* is!" The volume of her voice was rising and accelerating with each word. "She never even leaves money for Megan's food! I am sick and tired of this!" The volume of her loud voice scared Michael into tears. Seeing Michael confused and crying brought another fruitless sigh to her lips. "I just don't know what to do."

"You know, it sounds like you have too much on your plate," Billi continued, "Maybe the Social Service Department could help you with your problems taking care of Megan, and you could help them by answering questions about Michael. Nothing big, just a couple of things," Billi added nonchalantly, hoping not to scare her off. At that point, Betty Jo suddenly gave Michael a kiss on top of his head and promptly gathered her things to leave. The answer to that offer must have been "no." As she came through the door, I tried to engage her in conversation, remarking on how cute her little girl looked. She cut me off with a curt "she's not mine" and hurried on down the hall, Megan in tow, headed for the elevator.

A few minutes later, a flustered social worker arrived, disappointed to have missed Michael's aunt. While there, she took the opportunity to review Michael's chart, noting the numerous failed attempts to reach Sally Hedges. Because of the lack of contact with Michael's mother, and the aunt's apparent unwillingness to meet with her, she called the CPS office to let them know about Michael's impending discharge.

Our social worker relayed the cool and unemotional response from CPS: "Keep trying to reach the mother. We will provide education in parenting skills to Sally Hedges. A caseworker will be assigned to Michael and will assess the situation for possible signs of neglect. It is always our goal to reunite the family." Our social worker looked as frustrated as I felt, shaking her head as she left.

Family. What family? After the social worker left, I felt CPS needed to know more about Michael's situation. Trying my best to sound professional, and not angry and frustrated, I called CPS and gave a caseworker the whole scenario of the neglect that had landed Michael in the hospital in the first place. After all, CPS had the power to determine Michael's future. I had none. The caseworker just repeated their policy of reuniting the "family." It was like talking to a robot. I asked for a supervisor, but wouldn't you know, the supervisor gave me the same inane response as robot number one. Their directive was that if the biological mother came to pick Michael up, they would work with her in her home. "Home?" Hadn't I just told them that even Sally's sister-in-law didn't know where she lived? I hung up, feeling dumbfounded and more disillusioned then ever with the Department of CPS and their "plan."

10:30 a.m. T.C. to CPS. Informed them that Michael would soon be ready for discharge and we had tried numerous times to reach his mother without success. We stated our concern for Michael's safety if his mother actually did pick him up. EL/RN

All of us involved in Michael's care were shocked. How could CPS possibly believe the best place for Michael was in the hands of the person whose "care" had landed him here in the first place? How could they be so callous? What did their name "Child *Protective* Services" mean to them?

Still determined, I decided to drop by the CPS office on the way home. I climbed the dusty stairs outside the dingy, gray building. Inside the pea-green paint had started peeling around the dust-smeared window. Two lonely chairs sat in front of a vacant reception counter where a school bell had been placed, presumably to summon assistance. I heard voices filtering out from the inner sanctum, so I rang the bell. Laughter erupted, then fizzled down to mumbling blurbs. Could this laughter possibly come from the same people I had been trying to reason with earlier on the phone, the ones who gave only monotone negative answers to my questions? Minutes passed, so I rang again, this time with enough "vinegar" to knock the bell to the floor. Silence descended abruptly. Then I heard heavy footsteps coming my way. A middle-aged woman appeared a moment later. Her icy expression clued me in, before I opened my mouth, on just how far I could expect to get with her.

No introduction. No "Hi! Sorry I kept you waiting, how can I help you?" Just a cold "Do you have an appointment?" "No, not really," I responded, "I just got off work at the hospital and thought I'd stop by to talk with someone about the Michael Hedges' case."

"Oh did you?" She turned and bellowed towards the back room. "Anybody back there ever hear of Michael Hedges?" Some rustling sounds of shifting papers emerged in answer to her question. She motioned me to one of the seats saying, "If you had made an appointment, you would not be wasting your time or mine." I think it was hers she was most concerned about. I didn't expect royal treatment here, but things were deteriorating by the millisecond.

I sat in one of the chairs, as instructed, feeling all four bolts in the molded plastic relic from the sixties. Eventually, a case worker sauntered out and said "I'm Michael's case worker; you've got five minutes of my time before I check out." So I quickly I told her as much as I could about Michael's case and our concerns about his safety if his mother actually did pick him up on discharge. What I heard from Miss-No-Name was and I quote: "It is CPS policy to reunite the child with the birth parents. Do you need to see it in writing?" I left, the hot air buffeting me as I retraced my steps back down the stairs, feeling discouragement down to my bone marrow, feeling impotent with nothing left to do. Three days later Dr. Carrington wrote the discharge order.

8:30 a.m. Dr. Carrington in to examine Michael. Discharge order written. T.C. to Sally Hedges' message phone. No answer. CPS notified of discharge and inability to reach Sally. EL/RN

The morning crept along mercilessly, our team moving mechanically to accomplish our assignments. Phones were answered, food trays delivered, morning care given, medications passed. The sound of quiet expectation: deafening.

10:30 a.m. T.C. Another attempt to reach Michael's mother. A male voice answered. I informed him that Michael had been discharged and Sally needed to pick him up by noon. His response was "Good luck," as he hung up abruptly. CPS notified. Instructed to keep trying. EL/RN

I dropped the receiver back into its cradle. Keep trying, "Till when? Till hell freezes over?" Banging my head against the proverbial brick wall had given me a headache. Even so I could not keep from wondering, "*How* could CPS even *think* of allowing *that woman* to take Michael, even if she did manage to come for him? And just when were they planning on teaching her those precious parental skills?"

12 noon. Michael's mother has not responded to discharge order. CPS notified. They requested we give her until 6 p.m. If she hasn't arrived or called by then, Michael will be placed in a temporary foster home. EL/RN

Michael's caseworker at CPS had emphasized the word *temporary* reminding me once again that their goal still remained to reunite "the family." Who were they trying to convince? When I told my staff CPS's plan to give Sally until six p.m. to call or come in, anger erupted against the CPS system, against his mother, against the Social Service Department of our hospital, and even against Dr. Carrington (not that he deserved it). It just felt good to vent, even though nothing could lessen the frustration permeating our unit. With my own emotions raw, how could I relinquish Michael to Sally if she did show up?

For the rest of the shift, the usual chatter among the team members dwindled down to just the necessary exchanges. I picked Michael up, smelled his sweet breath, felt his heaviness in my arms. I remembered the whimpering sound of his first cry a week after he was admitted; he hadn't had the strength to cry before then. Next came his first tentative smile. Sitting down in my chair, I looked into big, round eyes which were now definitely a deep water-blue and felt the tickling fuzz of his strawberry blond hair. Kissing his forehead I handed him to Sara, who cuddled him for the rest of the shift. I wondered if some part of Michael would know, if only on a cellular level, that he was loved by all of us who had poured our hearts into caring for him over the last few weeks. I hoped so, with all my heart.

I made one last call just prior to the end of the shift to Sally's message phone. No response. What a dilemma: a baby ready to go home, but no family waiting to take him.

3 p.m. T.C. to Sally's message phone number. No answer. EL/RN

It seemed unlikely that Sally Hedges would be picking Michael up, yet the chance remained. Finally, the end of the day shift arrived. Our team had to leave not knowing the outcome of the drama in which Michael remained tragically and unknowingly involved. Naturally, no one wanted to say good-bye, even though we would send him off with hugs and kisses and a few tears on his head, knowing it wouldn't be any easier for the next shift.

Roger, the team leader for the afternoon shift, said he would call me as soon as this emotional roller coaster ride was over. At home I waited tensely by my phone. Finally, at six-thirty the call I had been waiting for quickened my pulse as I grabbed for the receiver. Michael had been discharged to a foster home. I gave a sigh of relief, feeling a weight lifted off my shoulders, though I felt sure there would be more to Michael's story. I hoped CPS would keep us informed.

The next day was too quiet on our unit. Our thoughts frequently turned to Michael. We knew we would miss him, we just didn't know how much. He was such a happy baby, smiling much of the time, bringing joy to our unit. Even the doctors hadn't been able to resist his infectious personality. The shift seemed to drag by, leaving us unsettled in its wake. The day was gloomy, even though sunshine streamed through the windows. How could such a little piece of life, unwanted by his mother, affect so many people and take so much from us when he was gone?

In the midst of the melancholy, suddenly Sara's face flashed with an idea. Turning to me, she asked, "What if Bob and I apply to be foster parents? Do you think there would be a chance we could get Michael?" I had no idea, but it wouldn't hurt to try. Sara's husband, a tall, unassuming man, occasionally came to have lunch with Sara and must have noticed how her face glowed when she had Michael in her lap. Maybe Bob *would* be open to the idea of becoming a foster parent even if it was a long shot that he and Sara would get Michael. I'm sure that over the next few days, Sara would give him all the good reasons she could come up with for them to apply.

After the weekend, I couldn't wait to hear how Sara and Bob's talk had gone, but I just had to wait. That Monday started off in fast-forward. Sara and I were too busy to talk until things slowed down. Some days are a blur of activity for the whole shift; I hoped this wasn't one of those. The admitting office needed two beds as soon as possible (ASAP). One bed was for Jeffery, a brain damaged 3-year-old with pneumonia. He has been in and out of the hospital since his near- drowning. At eighteen months he toddled out of the house and into a shallow drainage ditch. Undiscovered, his brain had been deprived of oxygen for so long that only mocking, jerky movements of his arms remained.

As soon as his room was ready, his mother, Maria, arrived with Jeffery. I always had a sinking feeling when Jeffery had to be readmitted. Not that he would die on us, but that he wouldn't. The only thing he had left was the brain stem activity that kept him breathing, but Maria still held out hope. She felt sure she could see Jeffery responding to her with his random movements. His doctor had been unable to convince her that Jeffery's neurological condition would not be improving. After we got Jeffery settled, she sat by his bed reading books, just as if he understood. Other times "they" watched Captain Kangaroo, Mr. Rogers, or Sesame Street. When Sesame Street came on, we *all* got to hear "The Wheels on the Bus Go Round and Round" so often that we caught ourselves humming along. An orderly placed a recliner in Jeffery's room, knowing Maria seldom left his side. It made me wonder once again, "Where is Michael's mother?"

The other admission, Mr. Riley, had cirrhosis of the liver secondary to his chronic alcoholism. This frequently landed him in our hospital. He always demanded a private room-- and not just any room--but room 135, the one with the best view. Mr. Riley had enough pull with administration to always get his request granted, even if it meant moving two patients to other rooms to make it happen. It wasn't hard to resent his arrogance in asking for this privilege and the hospital's willingness to meet his demand. The sound of a squeaky wheel broke through the normal buzz of our unit as patients were moved to accommodate this unreasonable request, reminding me to make out a repair requisition for that *stupid* bed.

After lunch Sara and I were at the nurses' desk. Telephones were silent. Doctors were back at their offices. It was momentarily quiet. I looked over at her, raised my eyebrows and said, "So?" Sara's face flushed as she told me that, yes, they had talked about becoming foster parents *and* Bob had agreed. Wow! Naturally, they wanted to be Michael's foster parents. Instead of fixating on that, they reasoned that eventually they would be providing a much needed home to a baby or child. This appealed to their desire to have a family *and* their generous hearts.

Picking up a still quiet phone, I dialed CPS, asking for an update on Michael. I was put on hold for what seemed like the rest of the shift. Eventually Haroldine came on the line. She identified herself as Michael's caseworker, telling me with a sigh that she had very little time for me. So

I quickly gave her our proposed desire for Michael, "My ward clerk, Sara, and her husband are applying to be foster parents." Silence. I went on to explain that because Sara had developed a special bond with Michael over the last six weeks, we hoped they would be considered first if Michael needed a permanent foster home. I added, "I'm sure you can appreciate the value of that bond."

Haroldine basically ignored my comments and said, "There's not much chance Sara and her husband would end up with Michael because the process for becoming licensed foster parents takes at least two to three months, sometimes longer." Then, in her ever-so-pleasant monotone, she droned on that if Michael ended up in "the system" it would not be in his best interest to be moved to yet another foster care home. Feeling spent, I hung up, hoping she was wrong, hating having to share this information with Sara. After telling her, Sara and I reviewed the conversation, looking for any positive note. We decided "not much chance" didn't necessarily mean "no chance at all."

Wanting Bob's support, Sara called and gave him CPS's disheartening information. To lift Sara's spirits, Bob, a man of action, wisely offered to go with her after work to pick up the application forms to start the licensing process. A smile crossed her face as she hung up.

We still missed the bassinet behind the desk, but over the next week we deliberately turned our focus to the steps Sara and Bob needed to take in order to become foster parents. We solicited letters of recommendation from our pediatricians. Sara and Bob got their blood work done on Thursday. Fortunately, Dr. Kraken, their family doctor, made time on Friday for their physicals. It didn't hurt that he knew of Michael's plight, and that Sara and Bob had to act quickly in order to have any chance of become Michael's foster parents.

The following Thursday Sara and Bob's modest, older home had to pass a safety inspection, the last step in the licensing process. The inspection was detailed, yet the findings were inconclusive. The inspector left saying he would have to run the data by his boss and then get back to them. Days of worrying went by. The following Tuesday, they finally got the call. The house was cleared. Final approval for licensing Sara and Bob as foster parents came in less than three weeks, a record, according to the Foster Care Agency.

With a knot the size of Texas in her stomach, Sara called CPS to inquire about Michael's situation. His caseworker, Haroldine, was in. Drawing strength from their new status as foster parents, Sara rushed to tell her that she and Bob would like to be considered as foster parents for Michael. Haroldine, surprised by the speediness of the process, cautioned that it was much too early for Sara to get her hopes up, emphasizing that Michael was still in a temporary foster home. She reminded Sara that the plan of CPS was still to reunite him with his "natural" mother. * Hearing those words once more drained the color from Sara's face. Uncertainty was the reality. Sara and Bob were ready, but nothing had changed for Michael. He was still held by a system intent on reuniting a family that wasn't! CPS was still preparing to return the victim to his neglectful, abandoning mother.

*As I am writing this, the department of CPS in Sacramento, California, allowed *seven* children in a recent year to return to abusive homes, ultimately leading to all of the children's deaths, according to an article by John Hrabe, featured in FlashReport (04/01/09). According to a report by the California Blue Ribbon Commission, the physical and emotional well being of the child should always be the foremost priority, not the preservation of the family. Another astonishing fact is that child abuse is the only crime where the state can reunite the victim with their abuser. For more on this subject see the web page of FlashReport or the archives of the Sacramento Bee that has been reporting on this CPS investigation. If you are passionate about this atrocity, there are oppor-tunities to volunteer with Justice for Children. To learn more about the organization visit the web site at: JusticeforChildren.org. In Michael's case our anger was ineffectual but our concerns were legitimate. I am saddened to find that the CPS system is still not fixed. How many more children must die before this issue is resolved--before the *child's* needs become the highest priority?

To cheer herself up after such a trying day, Sara decided to go to K-Mart just to look around. Her love of flowers drew her to the garden shop, but she soon found herself in the baby department. There were so many cute things to look at! On a sale table she spotted a tan and blue argyle sweater. It just happened to be Michael's size. She walked away, realizing it was too soon to buy anything. She didn't know when they might be getting a foster baby or child, and certainly not what clothing size would be needed. But it had been fun to dream. As she was leaving the department, the sweater caught her eye again. Sara mused, in the future they might get a baby the sweater would fit or she could always give it as a shower gift. The clincher was: it was the last one like it on the sale table. So she grabbed it and headed toward the cashier. Sara was relaying this as she showed the sweater to us the next morning. It would be hard not to notice that the blue in the sweater was the same water-blue color of Michael's eyes. It was undeniably cute, and I sincerely hoped she would never need to give it away as a gift.

By the middle of the morning, thoughts of the sweater were tucked away behind the needs of the patients, the orders to be transcribed, and phone calls to be answered. Dr. Carrington wanted assistance with a restart on Jeffery's IV. I went into the medicine room to see if Linda, my assistant and medication nurse, had time to help him before her nine o'clock meds. She did. Returning to the desk, I saw Sara with the phone to her ear, her face flushed as she fumbled through her words. "Are you OK?" I mimed. She nodded, continuing her conversation, "Yes! Yes!" She listened for a few more moments, responding, "Yes! Yes! We can do that!" The conversation went on for a few more minutes as Sara scribbled down some notes. Hanging up, she sat dazed. After taking a few deep breaths, Sara slowly shook her head in disbelief and said simply, "We get Michael!" as she sank back in her chair. Then with more conviction, her words wrapped in joy, she announced, "We get to have Michael!!"

Within what seemed like just seconds the team gathered around the desk, with everyone talking at once, eyes sparkling with joy, as Sara's story spilled out in spurts and re-starts. CPS needed the temporary foster home where Michael had been placed for another baby. Haroldine actually apologized for giving Sara such short notice and asked if she and Bob could possibly pick up Michael that afternoon. Astonished and still almost speechless, Sara picked up the phone to call her husband, then paused and re-cradled the receiver. She said "I think I'd rather share the moment with him in person. That is, if I can take the rest of the day off?" With tears threatening, I gave an affirmative nod of my head.

Patty, a nurse's aid and part-time ward clerk, offered to take over the desk. Without being asked, the team divided Patty's patients up. Then we ushered a flustered Sara to the elevator, making sure that the little blue and tan sweater went with her. Sara and I could talk later about mundane things such as work schedules. Even with all the excitement, the patients still received the care they needed and everyone was able to leave on time. Isn't it amazing what a little adrenaline, brought on by joy, can do?

When Sara called the next day, I expected her to request an immediate leave-of-absence, but she wanted to work the coming weekend to give Bob some one-on-one bonding time (on his days off) with Michael. She added with pride in her voice that from the moment they picked him up, Bob started calling Michael his "son." No amount of reminders about the unknowns for Michael's future deterred him.

Fortunately, Bob was comfortable with babies, probably from having a number of younger siblings or maybe from dealing with the baby animals on his farm. Consequently, "Mr. Mom" took over Michael's care for the weekend as Sara worked. On Sunday, Bob decided to venture out with Michael and take him to the little community church that he and Sara had been attending. The year before, they had asked the congregation to pray about their desire for a baby. Their friends there were surprised and delighted to meet Michael and to hear his amazing story. One frail, elderly gentleman haltingly approached Bob. He wanted to see the baby he had prayed for each day. Certain that his prayers had been answered, he reached out for Michael's tiny fist and planted a welcoming kiss on his fuzzy head.

Michael arrived at Sara's and Bob's home with very little of anything, so we planned a baby shower for the following week at my home. We were all anxious to see Michael again and to celebrate together. Friends started arriving early, even more than we had planned for. Every available chair in the house was pulled into service, and even then some of the younger guests ended up on the floor. It seemed that no one wanted to miss *this* party. Sara arrived a bit late, understandably, with Michael in her arms. Sara's mom, Michael's "Grandma," followed, toting the bulging diaper bag. At two and one-half months, Michael was the picture of health, making it hard to remember how that tiny remnant of life had looked on the first day I saw him. Lively chatter bounced around our great room. Stories were shared about Michael, reliving his remarkable journey. We were proud and amazed at Sara's and Bob's courage in pressing through all of the red tape, bringing us to this moment of celebration.

After everyone had a chance to greet Sara, she spread a receiving blanket on the floor for Michael and took her seat. Gifts towered around the rocker we had reserved for her. By now we were anxious to see what the carefully wrapped boxes held for him. Michael was soon snatched up, looking so cute in his new baseball cap (Bob's contribution, we were sure). We took turns holding Michael while Sara opened the gifts and passed them around to be seen, touched, and then tucked back into their boxes. Michael, all smiles, soaked up the attention. By the time all of the presents were opened, it was apparent that Michael's wardrobe needs were well taken care of. Plenty of toys and stuffed animals had been unwrapped as well. The last gift, from his "Grandma," held a hand-crocheted blanket in shades of blue, bringing "oohs" and "aahs" from the guests and tears to Sara's eyes.

We were enjoying the refreshments while Sara regaled us with a report of Michael's first week at their home. First, she shared her thoughts on the "joys" of night feedings. She hoped they would end soon! Then she reported on the challenges of getting out the door with an infant. There seemed to be an endless amount of "stuff' to haul around with her, not to mention how much longer it took to get her errands done. The mothers at the shower had no problem understanding what she was going through and shared some hilarious stories about the experiences they had had as new mothers.

Some of our guests reluctantly left early to be on time for the afternoon shift. The rest of us relaxed into quiet conversations. The late afternoon sun, softened by lace curtains, filled the room. In the dimming light I sat, trance-like, retracing the steps that had brought us to this day. Feeling the ups and downs of this emotional journey, wrapped in the moments of magic from the party, still feeling the warmth of the women gathered to honor the mother and welcome the new baby, this afternoon was just as I had hoped it would be.

Three weeks had scooted by since Michael had become a part of Sara's and Bob's life. Sara ended up taking only two weeks off, but cut back to a three-day week. Periodically, she stopped by to show off Michael. He continued to gain weight, and now had chubby cheeks and chunky legs. Most often he was awake and in a good mood, flashing his infectious smile. Thankfully, Sara reported that Michael now slept through the night.

Sara called in one morning on her day off and the distress I heard in her voice squeezed at my chest. Haroldine at CPS had somehow managed to contact Michael's biological mother. Now she wanted to set up a time for Sally to visit him. Somehow in our enthusiasm over how well things were going, we had let Sally drift from our minds. The concern about this development hung like a dark cloud over the whole unit. As our team commiserated about this development, our nurse's aid, Patty, reminded us that Sally had shown no interest in Michael when he was in the hospital (five minutes in the middle of the night didn't really count). "Why think she would come now?" Then she repeated that well-known phrase, "The best predictor of future behavior is past behavior." With that mantra as our talisman, we decided to assume that Sally wouldn't show up for her visit. However, there were times before the day of the visit that we flip-flopped between hope and despair.

Finally, the dreaded day arrived. The phone rang jarringly. Haroldine from CPS was calling to confirm the visit time, making it more of a scary reality. Sara and Bob sat on the couch, clutching each other's hands, watching the clock with adrenalin coursing though their veins. Michael slept in his room, unaware of the drama threatening his placement in Sara's and Bob's home.

Sally's appointment time came and went, leaving them emotionally drained and dazed, unable to move from the couch until Michael awakened crying. Almost mechanically, Bob hurried to get him as Sara headed for the kitchen to warm his bottle. They had escaped the "bullet." True to form, Sally hadn't shown up. Sara waited for another half hour to make sure she didn't appear on their doorstep, late and unwelcome. Immediately, she called our unit to share the good news. We could breathe again...but not for long.

A couple of weeks later the same scenario repeated itself with the same outcome. This soon became part of the ritual that came with being Michael's foster parents. Over time it seemed reasonable to expect we would get used to this. We didn't. Each scheduled visit created an intense feeling of vulnerability. One day it occurred to us that CPS hadn't called for over a month to schedule one of these dreaded visits. Maybe they realized the idea of reuniting Michael with his biological mother was an unrealistic goal. And then, just when we were feeling secure, CPS called once again asking for Sara.

Sara had gone to the cafeteria for her lunch break, so I took a message for her to call back as soon as possible. The familiar tightness in my chest returned, "As soon as possible," didn't sound good, but I was determined my face wouldn't show the concern. When Sara got back, I reluctantly gave her the message. Sara's hands flew to her face. "Oh, no! Not another appointment for Sally!" After she calmed down somewhat and took a few deep breaths, she reluctantly returned the call. But the call wasn't about that after all. This time CPS was calling to see if she and Bob wanted to take in another foster child, a 20-month-old toddler named Megan, Michael's older sister. Then they added that it would be best if Megan could be picked up as soon as possible, as she was in protective custody. When Sara heard this, she put a hand over the receiver and the news about Megan came tumbling out. Back on the line she told CPS she would check with Bob and call them as soon as possible with their decision.

It took a while for Sara to recover enough from the shock to call Bob. When she finally made the call, I *tried* not to listen in, but it seemed the conversation was going well, since Sara kept smiling and crying and nodding her head. The serendipitous opportunity to be foster parents for Michael's older sister seemed too good to be true. Even with this "out of the blue" news Bob instantly responded, "Yes!" Since Sara sat, still trying to compose herself and having little success, Bob offered to call CPS to tell them that they did want Megan.

In a state of shocked elation, I called the staff together, needing to share this exciting, jaw-dropping turn of events. We gathered in the team conference room and as soon as Sara could get the news out, the room erupted into sparkling showers of sheer joy. Immediately, everyone started talking at once. I knew that the joyful energy in the room would be etched in my mind forever. What an amazing day! A day that had started out in such an ordinary way. Who could have known? Once more we ushered Sara to the elevator, sending her home early to prepare for Megan's arrival. I took her off the schedule for the next week knowing we would talk later about when, or if, she would be coming back to work.

As the story came out, Megan's father had been apprehended for child endangerment when the California Highway Patrol spotted him riding his motorcycle on the freeway going seventy miles per hour while holding Megan on with one hand behind his back and steering with the other. Megan was taken directly into their custody and turned over to CPS for placement. By late afternoon, Sara and Bob had picked up a few things for a two-year-old and added Megan to their family.

The next morning Sara called saying she might need more than the three weeks she had taken with Michael to adjust to Megan's arrival in their family. "Might need?" I should think so! My own two kids were eighteen months apart, and I remember in exquisite detail what she would probably be facing. Naturally her request for a month off was granted along with the assurance that whatever additional time she might need, she would get. Since Megan arrived with only the clothes on her back, I asked Sara, while I had her on the phone for a date for a shower some of the staff had already started planning. To keep life in balance the good things need to be celebrated, and this certainly qualified as a *good thing*!

Ever vigilant, CPS continued making appointments for Sally to see Michael and Megan and she continued to miss these appointments. This continued parental abandonment *finally* rendered a ruling that Michael and Megan would be available for adoption. Naturally Sara and Bob wasted no time in applying for this legal bond for their family. Sally had the pre-scribed six months in which to demonstrate her competency as a parent for Michael and Megan to be returned to her care. So the six-month waiting period began. Sally occasionally made appointments to meet with CPS reminding us each time of the tenuousness of the situation, creating con-cern, even as we remembered that missing these appointments had been Sally's pattern.

Sara returned to work part-time after taking a six-week leave-of-absence. "Grandma" decided that helping take care of these precious babies was a perfect excuse for an early retirement. Sara sent pictures and came by our unit so we could rave over Michael and Megan and see how much they had grown. With their strawberry blond hair and little round faces, they looked enough like Sara to be her own flesh and blood.

Our unit had been busier than usual during the last few weeks. One morning Sara kept answering phones that seemed to be ringing endlessly. The sound of those phones and the overhead pages seemed to be running into each other like bumper cars at the fair. Too many hectic days in a row had shortened the fuses of our most easy-going nurses. I felt it too, the sense of being caged in by the endless tasks that sat stacked in front of me. Maybe it was spring fever. Anyway, I let Sara know that I needed a break and stepped outside our back door. The tingly fresh smell of the newly mown grass greeted me. I found a wedge of sunlight and sat down on the cool, moist lawn. It felt so good I wanted to stay there for a month or two, just soaking in the solace that soothed my flagging spirits and calmed my frazzled soul. After a few minutes of sitting in the quiet, I felt better. As I returned to my unit, a little part of me wondered if I needed to pursue another area of nursing. Maybe I should consider that later--maybe.

The months until the adoption proceeding seemed to be toddling, taking tiny baby steps. None of us could enjoy the joy and fun these two little ones brought without feeling a tinge of fear for the future. On the calendar hanging in the staff lounge we crossed off the days, bringing us closer to a desperately needed closure. Just two more months and the drama would be over!

When Sara arrived, a couple of days later, I noticed her face seemed to reflect both joy and concern. What a mystery. Hopefully, we could talk after breakfast. By then the doctors would be finished with rounds and off to their offices. This was a time when the unit often slowed, seemingly to catch its breath.

The day cooperated, providing a space of time to connect, so we grabbed some coffee from the staff lounge and found a small conference room vacant. I couldn't wait so I jumped in, "Sara, what's going on? Your face is a mixture of emotions I can't read." She sat looking off into space, still not ready to share. So I asked how the little ones were, usually a safe subject for mothers with babies. Then she burst into tears leaving me speechless. I sat quietly with her wondering what caused those tears that came so quickly to her eyes.

Then with no preamble, she said in an anguished tone, "I'm pregnant." Wow! How exciting! And this is bad news? After so many years of trying and knowing she and Bob wanted a large family, I didn't understand at all. Sure, it would be busy with three, but Bob was a great one to jump in to help. By then her sighs had turned to sobs. I hugged her close, speechless, feeling the next move was hers. As far as we knew everything was in order for finalizing Michael and Megan's adoptions. By now it seemed unlikely that Sally would come back into the picture. So what could be the problem? The adoption hearing should just be a formality. Finally, after about a dozen tissues and a few snuffling minutes, she started, haltingly, to share what was on her mind.

First she said, "I don't think you knew that before you came I had had three miscarriages. That was when I first started trying to get pregnant." This brought more tears to her eyes. I felt my heart sink in my chest;

so much this young couple had been through. Sara continued, her voice almost a whisper, "Then nothing for the last four years," as more tears fell silently down her blotchy face. "We didn't want to tell anyone until we thought I could carry this baby to term." Understandable. I had no idea. "So I will be five-and-a-half months along when we go to court. What if the judge notices? Well, really, how could he not?"

That was the fear. She went on to say that she and Bob were both worried that the judge might think that *three* children under the age of three would be more than they could handle. Or maybe the judge would think, since she was pregnant, the babies should go to a childless couple. At this point I started to worry, too. Logically I couldn't imagine that Sara's pregnancy would have an affect on the adoptions; but logic didn't ease my concerns in the slightest. So we hugged and prayed and hoped. She seemed to have gathered some courage from talking it out. Now it was time to get back to our unit and let the day draw our thoughts away from this unsolvable situation.

Two calls from admitting interrupting our thoughts. It had only been six weeks since Jeffery's last admission for pneumonia. He seemed to have less resistance to pneumonia and it was becoming more difficult to find an effective antibiotic for his infection. Not good for his long-term prognosis. On the positive side, new antibiotics were being introduced more frequently now. Part of me wanted him to recover, for his mother's sake, and part of me wanted him not to. He was getting heavier and heavier all the time. He was quite over-weight now, making it much harder for her to diaper and care for him. As the years go by, the future would be even more difficult.

The other admission was a cowboy with a rattlesnake bite on his leg, just above the boot line. He had a very cavalier attitude towards it (what did I expect, he *was* a cowboy) and I had a lot of curiosity about it, as it was a first for me. Even with the anti-venom he received within the first couple of hours, over time, the area around the bite sloughed off until a huge crater remained, requiring careful management. Frequent dressing changes were ordered to keep the wound from becoming infected. With the dressing changes came debridement (scraping away the dead tissue) until the wound started to ooze blood. Even though he was medicated for pain prior to these procedures, it had to hurt; but cowboy that he was, he never flinched.

Time goes by so fast and before we knew it, our calendar showed that it was less than two weeks before the adoption hearing for Michael and Megan. These days were scary--exciting, not surprisingly. Giddiness fringed with phantom fears. Finally the court date arrived. Sara had asked me to be there for moral support, but I might (Might? Make that would!) need some support too.

The Court House (nothing stately, not in our small rural town) was a single story, glass and gray block, contemporary building, with minimal landscaping. Arriving early for the hearing, I still hurried in to get a good seat. Good thing. The gallery was filling up fast, and by the time we were ordered to rise for the judge's entrance, there was standing room only. Usually a courtroom is respectfully quiet, but this time the babble of happy babies and the cries of tired, fussy ones were a welcome addition to the air that circulated in this crowded room.

As each case was called and the adoptions approved, deafening applause filled the room, the bailiff making no effort to contain it. The joy we all felt reminded me of the palpable exhilaration at wedding ceremonies when couples are pronounced "husband and wife." In both cases a family is being created.

Finally, Sara and Bob's turn came and they proudly stood holding Michael and Megan. The judge fumbled through some papers, then finally looked up: "Oh, are you expecting?" Sara just nodded, and I held my breath until the judge finally said "Congratulations!" He continued asking some routine questions, and then went back to look at the papers. (Oh, hurry, hurry, I was silently pleading). When he looked up again, he said "I find that the paperwork is in order. Therefore the adoptions of Michael and Megan by Sara and Bob Gladstone are hereby finalized," a smile crossing his face. Then he punctuated the decision as his gavel hit its mark. Those of us who had come in support of Sara and Bob stood, hugging each other and wiping tears from our faces. Despite the agonizing journey, another family had been created. A beautiful, magical moment, sealed for time and eternity.

The Path to Home Health

● ● ●

The Path to Home Health

● ● ●

IN THE MIDST OF A crazy shift, a call came for me from the corporate offices of NorthWest HealthCare Systems (NHS). I had heard about the organization, but knew no one employed there. Why did they want to speak to me? Ms. Whitmore, Vice President of Nursing, soon answered my question. They were looking for applicants for the administrative position in one of their home health agencies, located in a small community nearby. She said that if I were at all interested, I should send my resume to her as soon as possible. Surprised by this out-of-the-blue opportunity, I thanked her for the call, saying I would definitely give it serious consideration. Wow! My mind had been turning over ideas for a career change for the last few months. Maybe this was it! I promptly updated my resume and sent it, wondering what would come next.

Within the week Ms. Whitmore's secretary called to set up an interview. After I hung up, I felt tingles as feelings of excitement and nervousness vied for my attention. What if they *did* offer me the position? Was I ready to leave Station Four? On some days I felt like canceling my appointment. Yet, I would always wake up the next day feeling intrigued by the possibilities of this promotion, this step up the career ladder.

On the day of the interview, the two-hour drive took me through miles of peach, apricot, and cherry orchards, some in bloom, some still skeletons silhouetted against the sky. An early morning storm had blown through, leaving dark skies as a backdrop for the fresh, sharp, shouting sunshine. In one orchard the trees had been pruned so the branches fell like twirling skirts, their blossoms painted in the deepest shades of pink. Another orchard flaunted trees with branches billowing in white blossoms; a mist of yellow mustard ran down the rows, disappearing into the still-receding storm. Other orchards had white boxes scattered here and there, housing bees returning with honey in their footprints. Really, no matter how my interview went, the early spring show made the drive worthwhile.

At the corporate office of NHS, I entered a three-story reception area filled with giant ferns and other tropical plants, some reaching high overhead, drawn by the sun streaming through the massive skylights. Tall windows drew my eye to the plant-filled courtyard beyond. Not too shabby. The receptionist directed me down a tastefully carpeted hallway to a small conference room to wait for Ms. Whitmore. I sat anxiously awaiting her arrival, butterflies fluttering inside of me.

Ms. Whitmore, Vice President of Nursing, greeted me warmly, and then introduced me to Ms. Sinclaire, my potential boss, who would be joining us for the interview. Ms. Sinclaire asked me to call her Diane, putting me somewhat at ease. The interview started out as I expected, explaining what the position involved. Soon it turned into a lively discussion about health care in general. I came away feeling positive about the opportunity and the organization, hoping they were impressed with me as well.

Over the next few days, I thought a lot about this possible career change, hoping the position would be offered to me, and hoping it wouldn't be more than I could handle. When the call came from Ms. Sinclaire, I was offered the position and happily accepted it.

Leaving my staff after four years would be the hardest part. We were a closely-knit family. Our bonds had deepened with each installment of Sara and Bob's journey with Michael and Megan. After my final day of work, my staff surprised me with a farewell party. They wished me well in my new career in home health care. I bid my staff a very reluctant goodbye.

After a two-week break, I started my home health position. The agency had only been open three months when Barbara Salone, the current Administrator, decided to resign to be a full-time mother to her three small boys. Looking forward to my first day, I had arrived early. My excitement built as I waited for the agency to open. When the doors opened, Barbara introduced me to her staff with little enthusiasm. Maybe my excitement, eagerness, and expectations were unrealistically high. However, after spending a dispirited, grueling day learning the ropes from Barbara, I felt overwhelmed. Finally, I asked Barbara what she thought my biggest challenge would be: gaining the respect of the staff (when all of them, including the secretary, knew more about home health than I) or learning the regulations and scope of the business? The look on her face told me this was *not* the question to ask and that I would *not* like her answer. Barbara gave a negative shake of her head, a shrug of her shoulder, and responded that she had absolutely no clue. I was not sorry that it was her last day.

With no encouraging words for me, silence hung between us. Gazing around her office, my eyes fell on a group of framed degrees, certificates of accomplishments, and awards hanging on the wall. One popped out at me, a Master's Degree in Public Health. Perhaps her negativity was driven by a lack of sleep from being up with her three-month-old, or maybe she had had an argument with her husband, but I couldn't shake the idea that she thought I was not only a poor choice to follow *her* but that the job was way over my head. I went home missing my friendly staff, desperately discouraged, wondering if it was too late to get my old job back.

The next morning Diane Sinclaire from the corporate offices met me at the agency to continue my orientation. She arrived looking very professional in a cream linen suit, set off by a sage green silk blouse, probably calculated to accentuate her large green eyes and the natural straw-blond hair her Norwegian heritage had bequeathed her. Her welcoming smile and the warmth of her greeting eclipsed these external things. The sharp contrast between day one and day two could not be overstated. I began to feel like a "somebody" again. Diane, as she reminded me to call her, was probably in her early thirties, just a few years younger than I. Having her there, in my corner, gave me the credibility that I desperately needed with my new staff.

After chatting briefly with a couple of the staff members, Diane and I went into "my office." Inside was a huge desk that looked out of place in such a small space. Behind the desk sat a high-backed, *swivel* executive chair. Two generic office chairs, covered in grainy blue upholstery, stood in front of the desk. Diane waved me to the executive chair. I wondered how long it would take me to feel comfortable here, in my first real office.

Lynette, the secretary, offered to bring us some tea. We gratefully accepted. Diane wondered how my first day had gone. Wanting to sound positive, I answered that it had been a fine day, (after all I *had* enjoyed a great lunch) but that I was surprised that there was so much to learn.

Diane asked if I might be wondering how my days would be filled. Yes! Yes! Yes! And so it began. First she told me, almost in story-form, that NHS had recently entered the home health care arena in response to a wave of growth in demand for the services. HMO's and insurance companies were pushing for earlier discharge of patients from hospitals. Consequently, patients were going home sicker and needed follow-up care in their homes to prevent re-admission to the more costly, acute care hospitals. Home health care, providing a team of health professionals operating under physician's orders, filled that need by offering case management to homebound patients. Simple enough. I really appreciated Diane's starting at the beginning. It let me know that I wasn't hired for what I knew, but for the potential they saw in me. I would do my best not to let them down.

Over the next few days, Diane gave me an overview of the scope of my new position. There were numerous regulations governing home health as well as specific documentation requirements that I would need to be aware of. And, until the agency grew significantly, I would be supervising all the staff. There was an annual budget to prepare, strategic planning to do, public relations to be done with hospitals and physicians, and quarterly Advisory Meetings to prepare for and chair. Finally, as the administrator, I would be responsible for the hiring and firing of staff. My concern about what I would be doing from 9 to 5 was gone. Vanished.

Diane Sinclaire spent the entire week with me and continued to support and encourage me with frequent follow-up visits and phone conferences. After committing to be there for five years, I ended up staying almost ten. In that time the agency expanded from seven original employees to over forty.

As we grew, the first person I hired was Carol, a very young great-grandmother, to assist with billing. She soon became my personal secretary and stayed with me the entire time I worked there. Unfailingly cheerful, loyal, bright, wise, and with a strong work ethic, she was a joy to have. Carol set a positive example for the staff and helped to create the warm, friendly, family atmosphere our agency enjoyed.

George's Last Request

• • •

George's Last Request

• • •

GEORGE WAS DIAGNOSED WITH LOU Gehrig's disease (ALS) and became a patient of ours as this debilitating illness began to take away pieces of his life. When he became unable to breath on his own, he was transferred to a hospital in San Francisco that took care of ventilator-dependent patients. He and his wife, Hazel, had faced the progression of his disease with amazing courage and dignity. Now, George was near the end of the road and wanted to come home to die. Hazel called our agency to ask if we could take him back as a patient so she could bring him home. How could we *not* try to fulfill his last wish? Naturally his ventilator would be coming with him. Because he would be our first ventilator patient, (if we accepted him) a massive amount of preparation would need to be done.

The first step in assessing George's case, and by far the easiest, was contacting the discharge planner to find out whether *they* considered him a candidate for home care. The discharge planner spoke positively about having sent a number of patients home with 24-hour nursing care, including some on ventilators. She invited me to send a nurse from our agency to a team conference she would conduct with George, Hazel, a respiratory therapist, and George's physician.

I remembered being pulled in two directions. We could decline his case and avoid risking failure and damaging our agency's reputation. Or, being emotionally invested in him, we could decide to accommodate George's last wish. It would be a huge responsibility for us to assume. We needed a lot more information before a decision could be made.

We had just added Nancy, an experienced ICU nurse, to our staff. Naturally she was chosen to go to San Francisco for the two or three days it would take to evaluate George's case. She ended up needing four days. When Nancy came back, she was cautiously optimistic about the prospects of bringing him home.

Next, I called Diane to discuss the legal liabilities of this case and to ask for NHC's approval to accept this patient. Diane was pleased that we wanted to expand our services to include ventilator-dependent patients. She would need to run this scenario through several departments before making a final commitment. Within a few days Diane called and said that if we could meet all the protocols necessary and assure adequate RN/LVN coverage, NHC would support our decision. Scary good news.

Nancy became George's case manager. Her responsibilities were to set up the local services he would need: everything from selecting reputable companies to provide oxygen and ventilator service, to notifying emergency services of the highly irregular situation, and securing their assistance in developing a plan to evacuate the home and equipment in an emergency. The power company had to be involved to make George's home a priority in the event of a power outage and to recommend the appropriate size generator to meet his needs until power could be re-established. A hard-wired, non-electronic phone system had to be installed.

Then there was the challenge of interviewing nurses to hire and train to assure around-the-clock coverage. George's wife, Hazel, had to be trained as well so she could fill in for the nursing staff, in case of emergency. After several weeks the day arrived when George was brought home by ambulance. Amazingly, all of our preparations paid off and our home health agency had its first ventilator patient. Though he lived for only two and a half months, George got his wish to die at home, surrounded by loved ones. We felt a sense of gratification in being able to honor his request.

Bringing Jason Home

● ● ●

Bringing Jason Home

● ● ●

THE DISTRESS IN HER VOICE hit me before any of her words had a chance to be unscrambled. Brenda McCarthy had called our Home Health Agency and asked to speak with "the person in charge." I took calls from families or patients as they came in, if at all possible. Brenda McCarthy's call didn't fit either category, but my secretary knew I would take this curious call about a baby from his frantic mother.

Brenda blubbered out that her son Jason, was spending his first birthday in a large hospital in a nearby community, and she just *had* to get her baby home. Trying to calm her, I asked her to fill me in on her son's situation. "Has he been in the hospital for very long?"

"Yessss, since birth, and I want him home!" At this point Brenda's voice broke into sobs of frustration. I had been leaning back in my comfortable chair, but as soon as these words came tumbling out, I sat straight up.

"What? A whole year?" As I listened to her, part of me was thinking "How did I get this far in my nursing career without being aware of a case like this? I knew we lived in a small community, but you would think I would at least have been aware of a long-term hospitalization like this!" Tears garbled her voice as I tried to understand her words, hoping she would soon clarify her baby's situation.

Finally she took a deep breath and started from the beginning. Apparently Jason's lungs had not been fully developed when he was born a few weeks prematurely. He needed a ventilator. Since his birth, they had not been able to wean him from the ventilator. On Jason's good days, he wheeled himself around in his walker with extra long tubing to keep him tethered. He continued to be prone to respiratory infections. During these episodes he had to be confined to his crib to receive IV antibiotics. While this was undeniably a sad situation, I couldn't figure out how I could help. Our agency, like most others, was not providing pediatric home health care.

During our conversation I asked Brenda if she had spoken with Jason's doctor about bringing him home, the first step in *any* discharge. Her answer was "No, but don't you think a baby needs to be home with his Mommy and Daddy?" Well of course, but before I got the words out, Brenda jumped back in to tell me where she got the idea to call our agency.

She had seen the human-interest story in our small-town paper about our patient, George, being at home on a ventilator. She wanted that for Jason. Her request brought up memories of the extensive preparations done to make that possible for George. Thanking Brenda for her call, I promised to look into Jason's case, adding that she shouldn't get her hopes up. This was a very complicated request.

Yes, George had been cared for at home for over two months and things had gone well, but his situation was so different. He was terminal, wanting to *die* at home. Taking home a viable baby and assuming responsibility for his care 24-hours-a-day was an entirely different situation.

Later that day I called the discharge planner at Jason's hospital. She agreed to contact his physician, Dr. Jones, to see if she would be willing to entertain the possibility of Jason's being discharged in the care of nurses trained in providing ventilator care. She was unenthusiastically willing. Within the week, Brenda and I met with the discharge planner. First, we went up to the Neonatal Intensive Care Unit (NICU) to see Jason. He was a darling baby, arms flailing, bouncing up and down in his baby walker, obviously happy to see his mommy, and not at all shy around new people. How could I not agree to at least look into the possibilities of taking on Jason's case?

Mary Jane, Jason's discharge planner, offered to set up a team conference with Jason's physician, a respiratory therapist, a RN from NICU, and myself to explore the idea of bringing Jason home. The meeting was held. The team agreed unanimously that, in theory, the best place for Jason was home with his family. However, they needed to develop confidence that our agency could meet his needs. Understandable.

This hospital had never sent a patient home that needed a ventilator. Naturally, the team had many questions about how Jason's home could be turned into a safe place for him. Even though we had had one ventilator patient at home, the responsibility of caring for this baby loomed large. He wasn't coming home to die; he was coming home to live.

Many more team conferences were scheduled, and gradually the hospital team began to gain confidence in the idea of his home care. The largest stumbling block was getting MediCal to accept the plan. Its concern was about liability. It took four months for them to finally agree.

Once we had approval, we moved quickly to prepare his home. Our experience with George paid off; the plan came together like clockwork. Later that week Jason was discharged. The family celebrated with balloons, crepe paper streamers, and cake. Our agency celebrated as well, feeling the gratification of providing a way for a little boy to grow up at home. Jason needed our services for over two years. When his need for oxygen became rare, his family could manage his care.

Summer Takes the Reigns

• • •

Summer Takes the Reigns

● ● ●

LEAVING A SHIFT AT THE hospital for me was different from leaving the home health agency. At the end of a shift, hospital patients are left in the care of the next shift, giving a sense of release from duty. In our small home health agency we had only an on-call nurse for the rare after-hour emergencies. If I were away, the activities and concerns of the agency traveled with me.

This particular time the agency followed me to Lake Tahoe, California, where I had gone for a three-day weekend of skiing with a girlfriend. Prior to this I had only skied the bunny slope; Shirley had skied everything else. At forty-something, she said that I was too old for the beginner slopes so she spent the day prodding me to try one run after another, each one more challenging. I begged for mercy but she wouldn't hear of it. Finally, she took me to Siberia, an absolute cliff with moguls. My legs were already like over-cooked spaghetti. The only way off the mountain though, was down this run. She coached me all the way, but I vowed Siberia and I would *never* met again!

We got plenty of skiing in the first day, but the next morning we awoke to a blizzard. In the winter Tahoe's livelihood is based around snow. Now, it was snowed in. A freak storm had quietly arrived during the night. The national news referred to it as the "Storm of the Century." Lake Tahoe was paralyzed. All roads were closed with no estimate of when they would open.

My sore muscles sent me to the hot tub for a soak. While submerged in pillows of bubbles, the agency abruptly came to my mind like an abandoned baby. Could this snowstorm have reached our small mountain community, as well as Lake Tahoe? If it had, how serious would the damage be? A snowstorm, even thought rare, presented major challenges for our patients and especially for our nurses trying to reach them in snow-bound conditions. At an altitude of only 1800-2200 ft. our community was often advertised as being "above the fog and below the snow." Advertisements don't make the rules; Mother Nature does. And *she* occasionally sends snow, often just a dusting, but other times enough to stick to the ground and send drivers spinning in circles.

As soon as I was physically able to get out of the tub, I called the answering service for our agency. The line was dead. With the dead landlines, it was a given that the storm had hit our community hard. Digging out the cell-phone number for the agency, (new technology at that time) I called Summer, our on-call nurse for the weekend. Cell phone reception was spotty in Tahoe and in our little community. I was relieved when Summer answered. When I asked about the storm, she excitedly exclaimed, "This storm is incredible! It dumped enough snow to cave in the roof of Robert's Drug Store! Last night, large branches came crashing through some of the roofs of trailers. Oh, and power lines are down all over the community! I can't even imagine how many people don't have power!" Summer went on to tell me that she had already been pulled out of the ditch twice by AAA and it wasn't even noon yet. After the second trip to the ditch, she did let AAA install a set of chains for her. Thankfully! The last thing our agency needed was for her to be injured.

A snowstorm like this creates very real problems for our patients who are dependent on Meals on Wheels for food. The stakes were even higher for our two blind diabetic patients who needed daily insulin injections. Summer had triaged the patients and made a list of the ones that *had* to be seen. Then she called in a nurse who had a 4-wheel drive SUV to help make those critical visits. She was handling this challenging situation well. I was proud of her. I asked Summer to call me that evening so we could make plans for Monday. Normally, she would have been off. However, if the charge nurse was still snow-bound and I was still stuck in Tahoe, Summer would need to be in charge.

When she called to report, many of the roads were still closed and the power was off in most areas. Under those circumstances, I asked her to keep the agency going for another day. She willingly accepted the responsibility. Later when we had an opening for a relief supervisor, she was a natural choice.

Monday morning was cracking cold. The roads in and out of Lake Tahoe were open, but only with one lane in each direction. Shirley and I joined the other travelers, inching our way home.

A Portrait of Summer Scott, RN

● ● ●

A Portrait of Summer Scott, RN

● ● ●

SUMMER WAS A "LEFT OVER" from the flower-child era, each day coming in with a unique outfit. I once complimented her on her creativity in putting all the different colors and styles together. She tilted her head to the side and said, "Don't you know that all colors go together?" The agency's policy for dress was simple, but not defined. "Dress in a professional manner." Summer's fanciful outfits just barely met the criteria.

Though she was forty, Summer looked much younger. Occasionally, she even got "carded" at taverns. With her artsy style of dress and autumn-brown hair that fell halfway down her back, she looked more like thirty. Her buoyant spirit played into the "disguise," and made having her on our team a real plus.

Even though she was a single mom, she was rarely absent. When she was, it was mostly for her migraine headaches. So I was amused when the first call I got one Monday morning was from Summer *asking* if she could "call in sick." She readily confessed that she didn't have a headache, but was enjoying the great weather at the beach in Carmel with her son and boyfriend. They wanted to stay longer to see the Monterey Aquarium on the way home. Summer was willing to come in, of course, if I *really* needed her, but she would be about three hours late. She had a plan on how her patients could be re-scheduled if I would let her have the day off. Now what do you do with such a request? After all that she had done for me the month before during that devastating snowstorm, I gladly reworked the schedule and told her to have a wonderful time.

One evening, about a month later, Jane, the on-call RN, telephoned to let me know that Summer had been complaining about another migraine. This one was very severe. Her boyfriend had driven her to the ER at our small community hospital. Because her neurological signs were deteriorating rapidly, they immediately transferred her by ambulance to a trauma center.

Jane drove to the trauma center to be with her. Soon after she arrived, Summer lost consciousness. An MRI showed a leaking aneurysm in her head. She was immediately airlifted to the University of California Davis Medical Center (UC Davis) for neurosurgery. They tied off the vessel, suctioned the hemorrhaging blood, and drilled burr holes to allow her brain to swell in response to the invasive procedure. *This* was devastating news!

The next morning at the agency the air was heavy with concern. Everything seemed to be in slow motion. Conversations were muffled and tears shed. The staff members were highly trained professionals; none of them needed to be told of Summer's grave prognosis. Over the next few days, we would hear of a new procedure tried or of a change in her medication. Some days we hoped; some days we prayed; some days we just barely got through. Don Ashley, the hospital chaplain, came to several team conferences to help us cope with the gaping hole where Summer was supposed to be.

Several of our nurses made the two-hour drive to UC Davis, needing to see for themselves what this silent anomaly in Summer's brain had done to her. Many times we had been concerned about her migraine headaches, but for whatever reason Summer never treated them as anything but an annoyance. Occasionally someone would say, "You should see a neurologist about those headaches," but Summer would brush it off with a smile and an "I'll be fine" attitude.

Summer's desk was soon tied with helium balloons of every color and covered with cards from patients and friends from the medical community. For our agency, I went to our local nursery and picked out a coral-red azalea. I placed it on her desk, hoping against hope that someday she would come home to plant and care for it. That outcome was not to be. Still in a coma, she passed away about a month later.

The day we heard what we did not want to hear, I impulsively got my ears pierced, a rather radical move for someone from my ultra conservative background. I know Summer would have been surprised and pleased at the same time. Maybe I just needed a permanent reminder of the day we lost Summer.

Losing Summer was losing more than just a nurse. We lost the reminder that life is not about staying within the lines, but about letting our spirits soar, coloring outside the lines, pushing the boundaries, being in the moment, and squeezing as much as you can out of life.

Summer's body was returned to our community mortuary for cremation. We waited to hear what the family's plans were for a memorial. I was surprised when some of the staff came to me and said that she had no real family. *We* were her family. So we did what families do at times like these. Several of Summer's closest friends helped me plan a memorial service. The community hospital offered their Fireside Room for the service. We brought the azaleas we had kept at her desk. The hospital sent a large arrangement of red and white long-stemmed roses. Forty red helium-filled balloons bubbled up from the flowers, one for each year of her life, honoring a special request from her son.

We had known Summer for ten years. Although we had pictures and memories from our time with her, memorabilia of her first thirty years were non-existent. No relatives came to fill in the blanks. Missing were: a photo-board done by a grieving mother, a gathering together of the bits and pieces of Summer's life, baby pictures, childhood scenes, nothing showing her going through the awkward years, no images of her teen years or pictures of her emerging as a young woman, and finally as a mother with a baby of her own. No family floral arrangement arrived with carefully selected colors and flowers to reflect Summer's preferences.

The hospital chaplain gave the eulogy. For music, her boyfriend brought a boom box and played her favorite song, Roy Orberson's "Pretty Woman," giving a lift to the sadness that pervaded the very air that we breathed. Her friends told stories, both nostalgic and humorous. We alternately shed tears and laughter together. At the close of the service we took the balloons outside to release them, symbolizing a loving farewell to our friend. It was a riveting sight watching the China-blue sky draw them up. No one seemed to move as the balloons grew smaller and smaller in the vastness of the tree-fringed sky. I wasn't prepared for the emptiness that filled me when the last balloon floated out of sight.

The following spring we planted a ginkgo tree in the courtyard outside our agency. We placed a brass-plated plaque engraved and mounted on a granite stone, dedicating the tree to her memory. The ginkgo tree was chosen because it is a very unusual tree, and Summer was certainly a one-of-a-kind. Any other tree would have been too ordinary, unsuitable.

Summer's ten-year-old son and her boyfriend were the only ones outside the agency invited to the tree dedication. Her son showed up by himself, a sad reminder that he was truly *alone* in so many ways. He did seem quietly pleased that we were honoring his mother, but there was no sparkle in his eyes. We learned that he would continue staying with Summer's boyfriend until the end of the school year and then would be taken in by a distant relative. For me that may have been the saddest part of this tragic loss.

The Family's Role

•••

The Family's Role

● ● ●

SOME OF THESE STORIES ARE included to show how important it is for friends and family to be present to advocate for the needs of the hospitalized patient. With the nursing shortage that currently exists, it is more important than ever for an advocate to be at the bedside as often as possible to provide comfort measures and make sure the patient is getting the right care, the right medications, and the right treatment. Patients are vulnerable and may be unable to advocate for themselves.

Mom's Blood Draw Or"Just say No"

• • •

Mom's Blood Draw Or "Just Say No"

● ● ●

MY MOTHER WAS IN AND out of the hospital several times a year with pneumonia, a secondary result of her crippling Rheumatoid Arthritis. On this hospital admission her pneumonia was not resolving as soon as expected. This concerned me, so I caught the first flight down to Santa Barbara, CA, where she lived.

When I entered her room, a phlebotomist was standing at her bedside, looking for a vein, any vein, to draw a blood sample. From the distressed look on my mother's face, and the numerous band-aids on her arms, it was obvious this wasn't going well. Usually a very courageous and strong woman, tears welled up in my mom's eyes and her voice quivered as she told me this was the *tenth* time they had tried.

Nonetheless, she proudly introduced me as her daughter, a nurse. The phlebotomist looked up at me nonplused, poised to try again. I was furious. I told her to stop. She must have heard the not well-disguised anger behind my voice. She gave me a dirty look as she turned to leave, mumbling a derogatory name that trailed behind. My mother started sobbing in relief, so glad to have the torture stopped. In my mind I thought, "Anyone with intelligence would stop trying after the first two or three attempts." Her chart clearly indicated that the lab must send the best phlebotomist to do her blood draw. When any difficulty was encountered, an anesthesiologist was to be called.

At this point I rang for the nurse. Within minutes she was at my mother's bedside, chart in hand, assessing the situation as my mother reported her ordeal. As the nurse looked through her chart, she found an order already written to have an anesthesiologist start her IV for the administration of blood later that day. Both the RN and I immediately realized that an anesthesiologist could put a heparin lock in for the blood draw now, and then use it later for administering the blood. No one from the lab had checked her chart.

The anesthesiologist that came was kind, explaining that his own mother had Rheumatoid Arthritis. He placed hot packs on her arms to dilate the veins and soon found a suitable site. Then he used lidocaine to numb the area, inserted the needle, and attached a heparin lock, securing it carefully. He gave my mom a little hug before he left. Thanking him profusely, I breathed a sigh of relief. My tension and anger dissipated. I had become the "she-bear" for my mom.

"GJ's" Surgeries

• • •

"GJ's" Surgeries

● ● ●

IT WAS A SECOND MARRIAGE for my husband, GJ, and me. Each of us had children in their thirties, creating lives of their own, making us proud. Life was good. At our garden wedding, we pledged to stand by each other in various situations, including "in sickness and in health," but who expects "sickness?" Certainly not the two optimists exchanging vows that day.

First it was melanoma. A mole on GJ's back seemed to have grown. To ease my concern, he had it checked by his family doctor who believed there was no cause for alarm. A couple of months later we were visiting his daughter's family in the San Diego area. At the beach, his daughter, Suzy, pointed at the same mole that I had been concerned with, saying it looked larger than she remembered. That did it! I wanted a second opinion.

The new doctor said essentially the same thing that the first had. After this second opinion, I tried unsuccessfully to calm myself. With a lot of urging from me, that by now had turned into nagging, GJ agreed to have his sister's husband, Jackson, a surgeon, take a look. So the next time we visited them, Jackson looked at the offending mole. He assured me it did not look at all like melanoma, or any other skin cancer, for that matter. However, he would remove it for "cosmetic reasons" and for my peace of mind.

The following week GJ met at his office to have it removed. He called me when they were finished, saying everything about the mole looked good, telling me there was no need to have it sent for biopsy. That is when I put my foot down, saying, "Yes there is a need!"

GJ responded, "But honey, it will cost about seven *hundred* dollars!" As an entrepreneur, he had not carried health insurance for seventeen years. But I was adamant.

"There is no way I will forgive you if you die of melanoma, just no way, so have the biopsy done." As a result, the mole was sent for analysis.

Well guess what? It came back positive for melanoma, and there were areas where the margins were "not clear," meaning Jackson hadn't excised all the malignant cells. GJ had to have the procedure repeated, followed by another biopsy to make sure the margins were clear. He now has a three-inch scar on his back that I really like. It reminds me to follow my intuitions. He is *now* under the care of a dermatologist and receives regular total-body exams. What if I hadn't been home when he called to say he didn't need a biopsy? Where would he be now? Heaven only knows!

Within a few months, it was his prostate. Finally convinced that he wasn't invincible, he had purchased a health plan. When he went to his doctor for initial screening, his blood work showed an elevated PSA. He was immediately referred to the urologist, who did a biopsy. The pathology report came back that he had a "moderately aggressive," early stage cancer. Surgery offered the only definitive solution. He was scheduled for surgery within a few weeks.

GJ checked into the hospital very early on the day of surgery. I stayed with him until they wheeled him off, and then went to the waiting room. Having a family member in surgery is stressful at best. I had confidence that all was going well. After all, a well-respected urologist was performing the surgery. When the surgery went on for an hour longer than anticipated, fear gripped me by the throat, and objectivity went out the window. Every time the surgery door opened, I felt sure it would be GJ's surgeon.

Finally, I asked the volunteer to call the surgical suite. She relayed that my husband's surgery was taking longer than expected. Really, I *knew* that! No consolation there! Time was crawling by on all fours. Every time I looked at the clock it seemed the hands had only moved a minute or two. How do families stand this? Finally, his surgeon appeared looking confident, telling me that GJ had done well, but had lost quite a bit of blood during surgery. He said he would be making rounds that evening.

By the time GJ reached his room, his face was so white it was hard to distinguish him from the white sheet behind him! Lost a lot of blood during surgery? It looked like most of it had been left in the OR on sponges or in suction bottles! I asked his nurse what his vital signs were. His BP was 90/50! Why didn't they have the resuscitation crash cart in his room? The nurse said not to worry because that's what his blood pressure was in recovery. A post-op blood pressure of 90/50 might be OK for a patient with a normal blood pressure. But GJ's blood pressure was abnormally high, 150/90! I explained this to the nurse, who said condescendingly, "Yes, but he has just had surgery!" What a surprise! After spending five hours in the waiting room, how could I possibly not be aware of his surgery?

"Call the doctor," I commanded. No response from the nurse. "Ok, give me the number and *I'll* call him," as I reached for my purse and started the search for my cell phone. The nurse shot back, "I'll call if it becomes necessary." I responded, "With all the blood he lost in surgery, he is probably hypovolemic, causing his very low blood pressure. He may need a blood transfusion." The nurse responded, "But there are some dangers in blood transfusions." "Ok, but how does this relate to GJ? *He* has two units of his *own* blood stored in the blood bank in your clinical lab!" The nurse just muttered, "Really? I'll check on that when I get time."

Within the hour the nurse started blood transfusions. After the second unit, color began coming back to GJ's face and his blood pressure slowly rose to an acceptable range. I thought to myself, "I should be on the payroll here!" All this information was on his chart. But most likely, because of the shortage of nurses, it had remained there, unread. Most nurses are conscientious and appreciate family input. However, GJ's nurse did not fall into this category. Thankfully, the rest of his stay was uneventful and he was discharged within the week.

It has been six years since his surgery. His doctor does an extensive follow-up each year, and all the repeat PSA levels have been normal.

Lacie

• • •

Lacie

● ● ●

It was a cold and blustery Christmas Eve in San Francisco. My husband and I had been invited there to spend the evening with longtime friends, Randy and Judy. The warmth of their friendship enveloped us as they welcomed us to their home. The aroma of pine boughs and cinnamon surrounded us as we stepped inside. Their vintage home bloomed with Yuletide in every room. After introducing us to the other guests, Randy and Judy went back to their kitchen for the final touches to the meal. Guests trailed behind, drawn by the magical aroma. Soon, we were ushered to the dining room.

A narrow trestle table with long benches allowed just enough room for cozying up. Randy and Judy kept bringing mouth-watering dishes to the table. In the midst of these festivities a call came for my husband, GJ. It was his daughter, Suzy. I stood close enough to hear most of the conversation. Suzy and her husband, Paul, had taken their six-week-old baby, our granddaughter, Lacie, to Children's Hospital in San Diego. She was being re-admitted for a viral infection in addition to ongoing whooping cough. When GJ handed the phone to me, I could hear panic behind the words Suzy spoke. There was no doubt where we needed to be, and within minutes we were on our way.

Whooping cough. It's amazing how a whole generation can hear certain words and not have any emotional response to them. Those very same words brought fear to the hearts of previous generations. For example, my parents talked often about The Great Depression they had lived through. Their frugal lifestyle molded our childhood. How do you know what it really felt like to live through those challenging years? You don't. Stories reveal bits and pieces of the shards of reality that an entire generation experienced and remembered down to the cellular level.

My generation hadn't even been alive when whooping cough was a feared and deadly disease. For us, whooping cough was just another childhood illness that had a strange sounding cough, something we immunized our kids against, without a thought.

At three weeks of age Lacie had been admitted for whooping cough. We didn't realize how sick she was. When the pediatrician hospitalized her, we assumed he was just taking extra precautions. Lacie received excellent care and soon was discharged home. Suzy was instructed to watch for respiratory distress and signs of secondary infection.

Two weeks later Lacie went into acute respiratory distress and the pediatrician re-admitted her to the intermediate care unit at the Children's Hospital. The following day, Christmas Eve, Suzy and Paul realized they needed someone to be with Lacie in the hospital so they could go home, shower, and catch a few hours of sleep before coming back. That is when we received Suzy's call. If Suzy, a strong capable woman and mother, called for help, we knew the situation had become serious.

GJ drove, while I slept, and arrived in record time, five hours later. I didn't ask him how fast he drove. I did hear him joke much later, when the crisis was over, that the only thing that passed him that night was Southwest Airlines.

Suzy and Paul looked exhausted when we walked into Lacie's hospital room at four a.m. Their faces were strained with worry. Over the next several days, with the constant florescent light and activities going on twenty-four hours a day, time awareness blurred from daylight to dark. Lacie looked so tiny in the huge crib. She was getting oxygen and when she coughed ineffectively, her tiny airway was suctioned. She always fought this. Even though absolutely critical and life saving, it distressed me to watch the procedure.

Suzy had been immunized against whooping cough as a baby. It had lost some of its effectiveness over time. The persistent cough Suzy had at the time of Lacie's birth turned out to be whooping cough, not bronchitis. This answered our questions on how our little Lacie ended up with whooping cough.

At the hospital Suzy nursed her and used a pump to keep breast milk in the unit refrigerator to use when she was away. Because Lacie had a tendency to vomit her feeding, she had to be carefully burped both during and after each feeding. The doctors were concerned about her weight loss and considered starting her on IV's.

When I was feeding Lacie for my first time, and had just finished burping her, she vomited all over me. Tears started down my cheeks. I hated the thought of her having to be restrained for an IV. GJ picked her up and put her back in the crib, calling her nurse to help him get her cleaned up and to make sure she was OK. Her nurse was a tall young man. I still have a fresh mental picture of those two big men, hovering over our tiny Lacie, caring so tenderly for her needs.

Around the third day Lacie was doing better, so I was left alone with her while GJ, Suzy, and Paul went downstairs to the cafeteria for a bite to eat. The activity of the unit and the beeping of the machines were our constant companions. To be able to monitor each precious life, glass partitions separated the individual rooms from the nurse's station. In Lacie's room a tiny, decorated living fir in a small basket was the only reminder that it was still the Christmas season.

The baby in the unit next to ours had been discharged earlier that morning. As I stood there watching Lacie sleeping, I heard the staff preparing this room for another admission. Lights went on, curtains were drawn, and monitoring equipment was brought to the bedside. Soon I heard muffled voices and the footsteps of a family coming down the hall. Another baby was being admitted.

A little later, as I was watching Lacie sleep, I felt the tension in the unit begin to rise. Soon an overhead page announced a "code blue" for our unit. The wheels of the crash cart squeaked as it was quickly brought to the room. Voices of doctors uttered clipped commands. Then there was the sound of soft crying as the parents were ushered from the room. I could hear other voices, maybe someone from the chaplain's office, trying to encourage the parents that everything possible was being done. Time stood still, and yet moved on. Within the hour, the sounds in the next room quieted. Nothing more could be done to save the baby. The soft cries of the parents turned into inconsolable sobbing.

The parents were given as much time as they needed to say goodbye behind closed curtains and doors, but the sounds of their sobs could not be contained by steel and glass. In any hospital, there is an emotional letdown after an intensive yet unsuccessful effort to resuscitate a patient, but it is dramatically greater when the loss is an infant.

The mixture of emotions brought a swirl of conflicting feelings--so thankful it hadn't been Lacie, yet feeling guilty at the same time. I felt so sorry for the family who lost their infant. I wished GJ had been with me to help me find emotional balance.

When Suzy, Paul, and GJ got back from eating, I shared the sad story. GJ remembered seeing a young couple sitting in a deep windowsill with their tiny baby when they went to lunch. He said he even spoke to them, asking if he could find some chairs so they could be more comfortable. The young couple thanked him and responded that a secretary said a room was being readied. They said "We have waited quite a while; it couldn't be much longer."

Their baby had been transferred from a regular pediatric floor to the intermediate care unit. It is protocol to have a nurse accompany the infant and give a verbal report to the new unit. The parents didn't know how sick their baby was and how each minute counted. When help was needed immediately, the secretary went on an errand. A very sick baby and her parents were left in the hall. As the story was pieced together, it was clear that a tragedy had occurred inadvertently, yet just as fatally as if it had been planned.

As a nurse I felt conflicted. I *knew* there had been negligence dur-ing the transfer that could be compensated through the court system, but should I tell the grieving parents? It seemed like "ambulance chasing," violating their privacy, stepping uninvited into their grief. How would that ease their pain? What I really wanted was a "mulligan," a do-over, a chance for the hospital to do the transfer correctly. It may not have saved this baby, but at least they would have met the standard of care. Human error is inherent in the practice of medicine and does cause unnecessary deaths.

There is a prayer which says, "Teach me to care and not to care." Over my years as a nurse I have felt the dichotomy: wanting to care, a natural response, and not to care, an emotionally protective stance, and knowing it will always be a "two edged sword."

Shana

• • •

Shana

● ● ●

THERE IS A STORM RAGING outside in the predawn hours of this first week of the New Year. We have lived in Northern California since 1980 and this is the worst storm I have seen, heard, or felt. Rain is being driven haphazardly and almost horizontally against the windowpanes. Earlier, I heard our metal and canvas gazebo being blown over and twisted by the onslaught. Storms excite me, so here I am, sitting, mesmerized by the sounds.

What is it about this storm that is urging me to write Shana's story? I am not sure but I know I must. Shana and I met through our mutual friend, Anne. We clicked easily because of her sense of humor, independent thinking style, and our shared profession of nursing. She was 44 years old, mother of a 15-year-old daughter, Brenda, a 17-year-old son, Brandon, and a wife to an estranged husband, Trevor.

Anne, Shana and I thought going to thrift shops was a great way to spend a day. Shana was always on the lookout for vintage buttons, coins, or odds and ends to use to create her eclectic pieces of jewelry. These she consigned with some of the trendiest gift shops in Northern California. Her creativity was enviable, and I told her so.

How could Anne and I known that Shana would leave us within the year? Not willingly and not without a fight, but bravely and on her terms. A yearly mammogram had missed the mutant cells in one of her breasts. By the time Shana detected the lump, her prognosis was uncertain (even with surgery). There was some hope that radiation and chemotherapy would be effective in her fight against the cancer. At the least, her doctors felt it would prolong her life.

Her fierce independence kept her from allowing us, her friends, to go with her to the chemotherapy sessions, and kept us from knowing how much the fight for life affected her. Shana minimized the side effects she experienced and insisted that we not focus on her health issues. Period.

Instead of going on disability, for which she surely qualified, she took a position as a part-time nurse on the night shift at one of the local convalescent hospitals. She missed as few nights as possible as she braved the ordeal of the treatments. She had been doing this for over a month before she mentioned it to us in passing.

A few weeks later, Shana showed up with a wig she placed haphazardly on her head at times, showing the irreverence she felt towards her illness.

During this time, the San Francisco earthquake of 1989 hit. Our township, located four hours northeast of the disaster site, missed the jolt, but when the news of this disaster began trickling in, Shana drove down immediately. She offered her nursing skills to the massive effort of finding and treating the victims of this tragedy. She stayed there well into the second week.

The silent enemy pulled Shana deeper and deeper into its grip. Yet those of us closest to her were drawn into her denial and didn't see what lay ahead. One day Shana asked Anne and me to join her for lunch. We were laughing and enjoying her entertaining ways. Eventually, she maneuvered the conversation around to the forbidden subject of her health, catching us totally off guard. A follow-up visit to her oncologists and repeat scans revealed that the cancer hadn't responded as hoped, and had advanced, invading other parts of her body. Shana had an undetermined amount of time left. This news left us battered and bruised. Speechless.

As Anne and I sat dazed, Shana moved ahead with her agenda, planning her funeral. She asked me to be in charge of the arrangements. Maybe she thought that being a nurse somehow qualified me to do this. With no family except her children living nearby, she wasn't asking me. She was telling me, and accepted my stunned silence as consent. Next came her carefully thought out instructions.

Shana had picked a mortuary and already decided she didn't like the variety of taped music they offered. She would set a time with me to choose the music to be played at her viewing. The celebration of life service would be held at her church. Shana told us she had chosen the small youth chapel, instead of the much larger sanctuary, for a cozier atmosphere to accommodate the few friends and family members she felt would be coming.

Shana had even considered the flowers that would arrive and the arrangement for her casket. She did not like gladiolas. She asked (make that told) me to remove any that might show up in the bouquets. I promised that I would. Anne and I sat there, tears welling up in our eyes. Shana took a look at us and insisted we pull ourselves together so we could get on with the planning.

Our table had been cleared of our partially eaten, unappetizing food. However, Shana hadn't finished giving directions for what she called "the upcoming event." She ordered hot tea for all of us, and we listened as she continued. She had asked her estranged husband, Trevor, an expert woodcraftsman, to make a simple pine casket for her. Shana had gone by his shop earlier and reported that he had finished it. She was very pleased with how it looked. Anne and I sat there in a state of shock and disbelief, saying nothing. I couldn't help thinking "She asked *Trevor* to make her coffin?"

While we were recovering from that jarring bit of information, Shana took the opportunity to invite us to join her for a trip to the Napa Valley. She planned to take her daughter, Brenda, for a hot-air balloon ride. Anne and I nodded our consent. By now Shana was tired of our long faces and told us to "get a grip!" We finished our tea, gave hugs all around, and promised to get together again soon.

The Napa Valley trip, planned for the following month, seemed to arrive overnight. We piled into my car early Friday morning. As we headed down Highway 80, Shana told us she needed to stop at a linen shop in Walnut Creek. It didn't matter that it would add at least sixty miles to our trip. We were eager to make *this* trip, her trip, special in every way.

Shana directed us to a quaint shop. Its name, "All White Linens," done in old-gold English script, arched across the front window. We stepped into its wood paneled, lavishly carpeted interior. Subtle lighting spot-lighted the shelves, neatly stacked with white linen tablecloths, duvet covers, and bed skirts. Anne and I loved the shop, but wondered why we were here. Then we spotted Shana and Brenda over at a rack, notched into the paneling that held intricately detailed batten-berg lace gowns. She tried on a few and picked a lovely one with pearl buttons trailing down the front to the gathered lace at the hem. We didn't ask, but back in the car, Shana remarked that she had always wanted a batten-berg lace gown and planned to wear it at her funeral, sucking the air out of the car. Shana chattered on about the shop and the gown she had found. Anne and I had to agree it looked beautiful on her. Shana clearly wanted to go out in style.

By early evening we had arrived in Napa Valley and found our hotel. English Tudor cottages lay scattered amongst lush gardens. Anne, the raven-haired beauty, twelve years my junior, and I entered the spacious, elegantly appointed lobby to register. Henry, a young man with movie star looks, stood behind the ornate golden-oak counter. He nodded warmly as we approached and then turned towards Anne. He immediately started a flirty conversation with her, to which she demurely responded. When he finally looked over at me, he commented, "Oh, you must be Anne's mother," winning many points with Anne and none with me!

Following the map he gave us, we eventually located our cottage. The inviting interior drew us in. A cozy, wood-burning fireplace curved around one corner. Logs were carefully laid in the firebox ready to burn. More logs stood ready in a tarnished copper bucket nearby. All we needed was someone to light the fire. We each "had a go of it," without success. Finally, I called the front desk and shared our dilemma with Henry, hoping he could send someone to assist us. Within five minutes, Henry *himself* stood at our door, eager to help. I mused "How thoughtful of him," until he immediately turned to Anne and renewed his flirty conversation with her as he deftly lit the fire. What a surprise. Shana's much too young daughter and we "motherly types" were somehow ignored.

We talked well into the night. Shana's quick-witted humor entertained us, until sleep finally prevailed. Early the next morning, long before the sun was up, I drove Shana and Brenda to the field where brightly stripped hot air balloons were being readied for lift-off. The soft darkness began turning a buttery-yellow above the hills surrounding the valley, fading to a denim-blue in the vaulted sky above. Eastern hills, gilded in gold, announced the emerging sun, sending rays skyward and across the valley floor. In the early morning chill, paths of yellow flowers could be seen flowing between the rows of grapevines in the surrounding vineyards. The roar of ignited burners announced that lift-off time was near. Excited chatter of the adventurous passengers peppered the air as they waited. Soon the balloons were upright, reaching for the sky, seeming anxious to sail, yet tethered by ropes for the passengers to board. Caught up in the excitement, I stood mesmerized as each basket was boarded and released. It was not until Shana and Brenda's balloon sailed from sight that I realized I had observed a precious, unrepeatable memory. Tears blurred my vision as I found my car and retraced my journey to our hotel.

Back at the room, I found Anne *still* getting her "beauty sleep." After she awoke, we went to the dining room with its stately, mullioned windows. Stained glass panels diffused the morning light into bright rays of color. This ambiance lifted my spirits after the bittersweet experience earlier with Shana and Brenda. Our order of hot tea and Danish pastries arrived within minutes, served on a doily-lined tray.

Around noon Anne and I went to collect Shana and Brenda from the balloon ride. Their flushed and smiling faces told us that the ride had been magnificent. On the drive to Calistoga they excitedly shared the details, their words often overlapping each other. For lunch Shana had chosen her favorite Mexican café. The food was excellent, the service friendly, the décor authentic Mexican. I noticed that Shana had eaten very little, and ask if she was feeling OK. True to form she sidestepped my question. After lunch we wandered through antique stores and gift shops until we were all beginning to droop, time to head for home.

Two and a half weeks later, a surprising and deeply concerning call came from Anne saying Shana had been hospitalized for pain control. This was much too soon for us. Neither of us felt at all prepared for this stage of her illness. That evening we drove to the hospital together, feeling so much, yet saying so little. We dreaded having to face the reality of the ongoing march of this evil illness in our friend. We took the elevator to the oncology floor and found her room. She was still dealing with "the situation," as she referred to it, mostly with humor but this time accompanied by some pensive thoughts. On the way out, Anne shared how very difficult seeing Shana had been for her. I felt the very same way. Being a nurse didn't make it any easier to the see Shana, *the nurse*, as the patient. We drove home mostly in silence, sharing hugs and tears as we parted.

Several days later Anne called from the hospital crying. Through tears she said that Shana seemed to be slipping away. As quickly as possible I drove to the hospital. When I arrived on the unit, Anne sat slumped in a chair just outside Shana's door, telling me Shana had been released from the pain. Now grief fell heavily on our shoulders. Together we entered her room so I could say goodbye. Peacefulness surrounded her. I reached for her hand--it was still warm--but Shana was gone.

After a few minutes, we reluctantly left her room and took the elevator down. Fortunately it was empty, so we could just be with our thoughts. We were feeling dazed and unfocused. When we walked by the cafeteria, we stopped for tea, letting our minds find a few moments of rest. As we talked and shared memories of Shana, we agreed she had done life her way. That thought buoyed us as we hugged and parted in the parking lot for the drive home.

The day before the viewing, the mortuary called saying they were finished preparing Shana and asked if Anne and I wanted to come to see if she looked "presentable." How does death look presentable? We went reluctantly, not knowing what to expect. A somber staff member took us quietly down the hall to a room to see Shana. She did looked "presentable," but Anne, a beautician and esthetician, knew Shana could look much better. We left saying we would return to make some adjustments. We were soon back with Anne's supplies and she began to work her magic. She applied natural looking make-up and lipstick in just the right shades to accentuate Shana's lovely features. Her hair was next. When Anne finished, Shana wasn't just "presentable," she was beautiful, looking rested and comfortable in her lovely white gown. Somehow, tending to Shana provided an unexpected measure of comfort for us.

Shana had picked music by Enya for her viewing. We tucked a player amongst the flowers, minus *any* gladiolas, just as she had requested, even though the mortician frowned on this. The sheen of her varnished pine casket reflected the subtle lighting in the room, filled with the fragrance of the flowers and the soft music. Anne and I knew Shana would be pleased with how everything she had chosen for this service came together, creating a serene environment for her family and her many friends.

The next morning dawned cool and clear. Shana had been wrong about not needing a larger space for the memorial. All the seats were filled in the Youth Chapel long before the service started. Chairs were brought into the foyer and quickly filled. More friends lined the walls of the chapel. The celebration of life service was simple and beautiful. Somehow her daughter, Brenda, had the strength to sing with the youth choir, which shouldn't have surprised us, as she *was* her mother's daughter. Shana's pastor gave a moving eulogy, and then it was time to close her casket. Shana, being a bit a feminist, had requested that four of her girlfriends join Anne and me as pallbearers. A brief graveside service for family and her closest friends took place at the century old cemetery just up the hill from the church. After the pastor said a few words and a prayer, each of us tossed a flower onto her casket as it was lowered gently into the warm and waiting earth. Shana will always live in our hearts, her laughter will ring in our ears, and her spirit will inspire us to live life well, and on our own terms.

When the Wind Blows

• • •

When the Wind Blows

● ● ●

I HAD ALWAYS WANTED MORE than two children: three, maybe even four. My husband agreed that three or four would be fine; after all, he was the oldest of four. We would have two close together, and then another one or two a few years later. So, when our first two were ten and twelve, the time seemed right to add the next addition to our family.

Soon a third baby was expected! My last two pregnancies had been easy. And this one seemed to be on the same track, no nausea or vomiting, just a little tiredness. I had friends who weren't so lucky. One swears her morning sickness lasted all day and that she even vomited on the way to the delivery room! Pregnancy seemed to suit my body and I had never felt better.

Three or four weeks later I was teaching nursing students in the skills lab at the local junior college. It was late one Friday afternoon when I felt a sharp pain in my right lower abdomen. Thinking it might be just gas, I took some slow deep breaths as I continued to teach. That didn't help, in fact the pain was getting worse with each breath.

Finally excusing myself, I headed upstairs to the nursing office to let them know I needed to go home. Then I called my OB-GYN doctor and told the receptionist about my pain and that I thought it was from an ectopic pregnancy. She asked me to hold. Soon Dr. St. Claire picked up the line and started asking questions about my symptoms. Then he paused for a few moments. Over the phone it sounded like he was reviewing my chart. When he came back on the line, he said the pain was probably normal, suggesting that maybe I had forgotten what it was like to be pregnant. He did recommend I go home, get some rest, and call him later if it became necessary.

I obviously already *thought* it was necessary or I wouldn't have bothered to call him. Hanging up the phone left me feeling frustrated, wishing he had just told me to come by his office. That would have eased my overly active imagination.

By now the pain was distracting enough that I was bending over, holding my abdomen. The nursing department staff wanted to call an ambulance for me, but that didn't seem necessary. Driving myself home was probably not a viable option, so I called my husband. He was there in a just a few minutes to get me and help "ease" me into his *little* Triumph; I hadn't thought that one out very well. Don was as perplexed and concerned as I was. At home, he drew a bath for me while I sat doubled over on the toilet. The warm bath did ease the pain somewhat. Don helped me out of the tub and to our bed.

Soon the pain had increased back to its original level. I hated to call my doctor again. After all it was a Friday evening, the office was closed, and the answering service would have to page him.

I didn't want to disturb him if it really was nothing to worry about. I called my brother-in-law, an internist, instead. He came to our house from a party that he and my sister had been enjoying with friends.

He decided that the intensity of the pain needed to be evaluated at the emergency room. I didn't want to get out of bed, wishing somehow to just magically arrive there, without having to move. It didn't happen that way, of course. He and Don helped me, as carefully as they could, down the flight of stairs and into his car. Thank goodness, at least he had a full-sized car for the trip to the hospital.

On arrival, the ER doctor took a brief history and called my OB-GYN to come in to see me. As soon as Dr. St. Claire arrived, he reviewed my admission vitals, examined me, and ordered a sonogram. A white circle of light that the technician pointed out to me, confirmed my pregnancy. The picture on the screen was inconclusive about whether or not things were progressing normally. This was in 1980 and sonogram technology was fairly new, but I could have told them that something *was* wrong.

I was admitted to the hospital for observation and pain management. My doctor ordered vital signs to be taken every two hours, had an IV started, and just in case I would need surgery later, didn't allow me food or fluids.

Feeling braver after being settled in bed, and with the pain medication making me drowsy, I told my husband he should go home and be with the kids for the night. He asked if I was sure. I responded jokingly, "Oh yes, after all, I am a nurse. I'll be OK." My doctor had given me some hope that what I was experiencing might not be related to my pregnancy, and that gave me something to hold on to. By morning we would know more.

It would be nice to tell you that as a nurse I was the perfect patient, but as soon as I was alone in my room, I started to worry. What if it *was* an ectopic pregnancy? What if I died of internal hemorrhaging in my sleep? After all they had given me something for pain and as a very sound sleeper, I could sleep through almost anything--maybe even dying!

Not wanting to let the nursing staff know of my fears, I decided to use my own nursing knowledge to monitor myself. Checking my pulse seemed like a good place to start but, of course, my nurses' watch was at home. Not to worry, I would count sixty seconds! A thousand and one, a thousand and two... How I thought I could count my pulse while counting the seconds, I'll never know. Maybe the pain medication was marring my thinking. My pulse was faster than the sixty seconds I counted, but it wasn't racing, so I figured I wasn't going into shock. You may have heard the expression that if a doctor decides to treat himself, he has a fool for a patient. I suspect that goes for nurses as well, but at the time my plan *seemed* reasonable.

Someone had closed my door to insure my room was quiet, since it was located almost directly across from the nurses' station. It was a nice gesture, but my anxiety level went up, as I lay there wide-awake, still imagining that I could die in the night and no one would know.

I was getting really sleepy by now, but instead of relaxing, I decided that getting sleepy might mean I was dying from blood loss. I tried to calm myself by saying the Twenty-Third Psalm, and was doing okay until I got to the part about "Yea, though I walk through the valley of the shadow of death," then I panicked. Enough of this self-monitoring stuff! After all, my insurance was paying for me to be here and to be carefully monitored by nurses!

I rang my bell. A nice male nurse was immediately at my bedside, and I sheepishly told him my fears and asked him to take my blood pressure again, even though I knew it wasn't due again for another hour. He was kind and reassuring and re-took my vitals, telling me everything was normal. Then I needed to go to the bathroom and he asked if I wanted him to get a female nurse to help me. I thought to myself, "Now that I know I'm not dying, what else mattered?"

Well, there was the problem of the hospital gown with no back, which he was kind enough to hold together for me as he steadied my gait, opened the bathroom door, and wheeled the IV stand in with me.

He partially closed the door "for privacy," and stood outside to make sure I was okay. This, I had somehow not anticipated. Being quite modest, and a little more alert after the walk to the bathroom, the idea of a female nurse was sounding better all the time. Too late for that this time. He was discrete and professional. After thinking about it, if I was comfortable with a male physician, why not a male nurse? After settling me in, he asked if I'd like the door left open, a bit. I willingly accepted, feeling safe, like a child with a night-light.

I awoke the next day with a phlebotomist gently telling me they needed more blood for lab work. Through my foggy medicated haze, I could see that it was still dark outside! What was the rush? As a patient I was beginning to learn that I was not really in control, my doctor's orders and the staff's routines were. I took my arm out from under my warm covers and she got what she came for--more of my blood. It's probably a good thing for nurses to be the patient, and, at least once, to see things from the other side of the bed.

When my doctor came by later on his morning rounds, he said that the results of my lab indicated that my situation was deteriorating and they would need to do surgery right away. Deteriorating? Wasn't there a less scary word to use? I asked him what he meant, and he replied that my hemoglobin had dropped and I was bleeding internally. They needed to do an exploratory operation to find out what was causing the problem. He needed me to sign a consent form that I was more than willing to do.

The problem did turn out to be an ectopic pregnancy that was leaking, but hadn't fully ruptured. Now if he had just listened to me in the first place. By late afternoon, visitors were coming to see me. All of us were relieved that they had caught the ectopic pregnancy in time and that I had survived. Each post-op day was better, my body was healing, and I was soon discharged home.

It was so good to be back in my own bed, with a private nurse, my dear grandmother. The mail brought get-well cards and among them was one from my friend, a medical social worker. On the inside she had added, "I am thankful that you survived the ordeal of emergency surgery, but sorry about the loss of your baby." Her thoughtful words stopped me short. Tears stung my eyes and dripped down my cheeks. After reading her card, I closed my eyes and could see the full moon of a glow on the sonogram that was the life that was growing in me. Even though it had gotten stuck in my tube, it was a baby, our baby. Everything the baby would have been was there at the moment of conception. The baby's genetic code included its gender, its intellectual potential, its personality, the color of its hair and eyes, even that dimpled chin. And at six weeks of age its little heart would have started beating. Our baby's due date was already circled on the calendar. Names had been running through my mind. Bradley, for a boy, after a darling little six-year-old boy who was a patient of mine. Emily, for a girl. I sat there reflecting on my friend's card. The healing of my heart had begun.

CPR in Church

• • •

CPR in Church

• • •

"ANNIE," THE DEMONSTRATION DOLL USED for CPR certification, had been "rescued" by me numerous times as part of certification renewal. As a lab instructor, I had even taught CPR many times to nursing students. What I had never done is actually perform CPR on a real human, anywhere, ever. Yes, I had observed CPR a number of times over the years. I had even assisted with drawing up medications and handing them to the people who were performing CPR. But actually *doing* the chest compressions or *giving* mouth-to-mouth resuscitation? Never.

One day during a church service, an opportunity came for me to observe, up close and personal, a gentleman who needed this procedure. Even though the church held over a thousand attendees, it seems that, as creatures of habit, we keep going back to "our pew" week after week, creating a familiarity with the people sitting around us. I recognized a few doctors and nurses who sat in "my" section, the right front quarter.

We were kneeling on the padded benches, which came in handy when the pastoral prayer got a bit lengthy, which it often did. The pastor was just getting into his prayer when I heard a little rustling and someone very quietly asking "Is there a doctor in the house?" If they really needed one, unless God passed the message on, no one was going to hear it or respond to it. I looked up and a man, three pews up and a little to my left, was turning purple! This man was dying before my eyes! Without even thinking I jumped up and "called a code" in a loud voice, "I need help with CPR! SOMEONE CALL 911!

Immediately an ER doctor and two ICU nurses materialized from our corner of the church. The man was moved to the aisle, giving space for the doctor and nurses to begin CPR. It wasn't until then that I recognized the man, Mr. Dare, a long-time church member.

Mr. and Mrs. Dare were active in the church and enjoyed spending their retirement with their nearby grandchildren and traveling. His wife came to stand by me, tears falling, and fear palatable around her. Her first words were "I can't lose him, I've already lost two husbands!"

I put my arms around her and said, "Well, you are *not* going to lose this one," with more conviction than I felt. CPR continued and within a very few minutes he started to respond as color came back to his face. I can't pretend to tell you how grateful I felt, because in my years as a hospital nurse I had never actually observed a successful CPR. The paramedics arrived with a gurney and quietly wheeled him out, as the ER physician followed alongside.

By now the preacher was finally finishing his scripted prayer, without any interruption or mention of this dramatic event. I guess he felt that "The show must go on." I later learned that Mr. Dare had experienced a cardiac conduction disorder. Because of the quick response of the CPR team, he had no cerebral deficits. His doctor implanted a pacemaker, and within days he was discharged from the hospital. He and his wife were given fifteen more years of quality life together. On seeing his obituary in the church paper, my mind took me back to that day. Every detail came back, especially the sense of amazement and absolute joy I felt knowing he had survived. Good Happens.

Dear Reader,

Your Patient Stories Are Needed

Because my heart goes out to children with devastating illness, St. Jude's Children's Research Hospital will receive a portion of the royalties from this book.

For comments about this book or to submit a story for consideration, please contact me at: Heart-Beats@att.net and we are on <u>Facebook</u> as well as Heart Beats. We'd like you to "like us" on <u>Facebook.</u>

Thank you,
Evelyn

ACKNOWLEDGMENTS

My sincerest appreciation goes TO my husband G'ert Jonsson, who has encouraged my creative writing when my spirits flagged. Thank you to Jean Hardt Mertz, RN BSN my friend who suggest that I "should" write a book. A huge measure of gratitude must go to my friend, Jan Kirby, MA, a English professor who has worked tirelessly providing massive amounts of editorial assistance. Thank you to readers of the manuscript who provided helpful suggestions: Norma Rice, RN, Patricia Davis, RN, and to a budding editor, at sixteen, Amanda Priest.

www.ingramcontent.com/pod-product-compliance
Lightning Source LLC
Chambersburg PA
CBHW070226190526
45169CB00001B/95